THE MAUDSLEY

Maudsley Monographs

MAUDSLEY MONOGRAPHS

HENRY MAUDSLEY, from whom the series of monographs takes its name, was the founder of The Maudsley Hospital and the most prominent English psychiatrist of his generation. The Maudsley Hospital was united with the Bethlem Royal Hospital in 1948, and its medical school, renamed the Institute of Psychiatry at the same time, became a constituent part of the British Postgraduate Medical Federation. It is now associated with King's College, London, and entrusted with the duty of advancing psychiatry by teaching and research. The Bethlem-Maudsley NHS Trust, together with the Institute of Psychiatry, are jointly known as The Maudsley.

The monograph series reports work carried out at The Maudsley. Some of the monographs are directly concerned with clinical problems; others, less obviously relevant, are in scientific fields that are cultivated for the furtherance of psychiatry.

Maudsley Monographs number thirty-six

Delusions

Investigations into the Psychology of Delusional Reasoning

Philippa A. Garety, MA, MPhil, PhD,
FBPsS, CPsychol

*Professor of Clinical Psychology, United Medical and Dental Schools of
Guy's and St. Thomas' Hospitals, University of London, formerly Senior
Lecturer in Psychology, Institute of Psychiatry and Honorary Consultant
Clinical Psychologist, Bethlem Royal and Maudsley Trust*

David R. Hemsley, MA, MPhil, PhD, FBPsS, CPsychol
*Professor of Abnormal Psychology, Institute of Psychiatry and Honorary
Consultant Clinical Psychologist, Bethlem Royal and Maudsley Trust*

Psychology Press
An imprint of Erlbaum (UK) Taylor & Francis

First published in hardback by Oxford University Press, 1994

Reprinted in paperback 1997

Psychology Press Ltd., Publishers
27 Church Road
Hove
East Sussex, BN3 2FA
UK

British Library Cataloguing in Publication Data

A catalogue record for this book is available from the British Library

   ISBN 0-86377-785-6
   ISSN 0076-5465

Printed and bound in the United Kingdom by Biddles Ltd., Guildford & Kings Lynn

Preface

Delusions have relatively rarely been the subject of empirical research, despite their importance as key symptoms of psychosis. This is in part because the syndrome of schizophrenia rather than individual symptoms has captured the attention of many workers and in part because delusions, as private mental phenomena, are not well suited to purely observational or behavioural methods of enquiry. For the past two decades, however, cognitive psychology has been in its ascendancy and delusions, as beliefs, are particularly amenable to investigation applying cognitive concepts and methods. With such an approach it is possible to consider continuities between delusional and ordinary beliefs, as well as to seek to identify differences. The work presented here employs this neglected strategy of single-symptom research and the tools of cognitive psychology.

This monograph consists of a series of studies of delusions, parts of which formed a PhD thesis awarded to P.A.G. by the University of London in 1990. The monograph otherwise draws on published work of the joint authors and our collaborators at the Institute of Psychiatry, Jane Brett-Jones, Farzeen Huq, Brian Everitt, and Simon Wessely. The remainder of the text offers some of our more recent thoughts on this complex subject.

London   P.A.G.
July 1994   D.R.H.

Acknowledgements

This monograph describes work conducted over a decade and innumerable people have helped us in some way. Although we cannot name them all, we would like to thank some people especially.

Firstly, we are grateful for the forebearance shown by the many people with delusions who answered our questions, filled out our forms, and underwent our tests. They did not benefit directly from our endeavours; we hope that this work will make some contribution to the alleviation of the suffering of people with similar problems. The studies were all conducted at the Bethlem Royal and Maudsley Hospitals and a Special Hospital. The medical and nursing staff of these hospitals were generous with their time in helping to identify suitable patients and in providing information.

Statistical guidance was given by Graham Dunn, Brian Everitt, and Graham Robertson. A number of colleagues and students collaborated in certain studies, in particular Jane Brett-Jones, Farzeen Huq, and Simon Wessely.

Finally, the clinical psychology secretariat at the Institute of Psychiatry has been our base throughout this time. The secretaries have unfailingly supported us, both professionally and emotionally. Our particular thanks go to Moira Hall, who has undertaken the demanding task of preparing this manuscript.

Contents

Tables

Figures

1 Concepts of delusion

INTRODUCTION

This book is about delusion, the psychiatric symptom which, for many, epitomizes madness. It is extremely common, and is present in a wide variety of conditions (Maher and Ross 1984). Definitions have, until recently, achieved a broad consensus within psychiatry (although they pose widely acknowledged social and political difficulties (Moor and Tucker 1979)). Standard definitions generally incorporate a proposition, explicit or implicit, concerning the irrationality of delusional beliefs. In this book, we propose that accepted concepts of delusions are inadequate, that the model of rationality they embody is outmoded, and that the reasoning of people with delusions is sometimes abnormal, but not in the way generally thought. Evidence will be presented to support this argument from reviews of existing literature and with data from four original studies.

DEFINITIONS

Many have written of delusion without attempting to define it (for example Arthur 1964), perhaps considering the dictionary definition sufficient: 'a fixed false opinion with regard to objective things, especially as a form of mental derangement' (*Shorter OED*, first found with this meaning in 1552). This concisely embraces the central characteristics of modern psychiatric definitions, which themselves derive from the work of the German phenomenologists of the late nineteenth and early twentieth centuries, among them Kraepelin (1899), Bleuler (1911) and, most importantly, Jaspers (1913).

Jasperian concepts

Jaspers begins his essay 'Delusion and awareness of reality' by stating that 'to say simply that a delusion is a mistaken idea is firmly held by the patient and which cannot be corrected is superficial and incorrect. A delusion is a primary phenomenon — experiencing and thinking that something is real: this constitutes a transformation of one's total awareness of reality.' Jaspers is regarded (for example Schmidt 1940) as having made a breakthrough in the understanding of delusions by distinguishing, according to psychological criteria, between two classes of delusional ideas:

Some can be understood in the light of related affect, other experiences, hallucinations . . . others are not amenable to further psychological analysis but are phenomenologically irreducible. The former we call delusion-like ideas, the latter genuine delusional ideas . . . We would describe as genuine delusional ideas only those which have their manifest source in a primary pathological experience, or can be explained only in terms of a personality change. (Quoted by Schmidt 1940, p. 105)

This distinction between 'primary' and 'secondary' delusions has been extremely influential in psychiatry, although it continues to lack an empirical basis.

Delusions, Jaspers holds, are characteristically

(1) held with extraordinary conviction, with an incomparable subjective certainty;

(2) maintained imperviously to other experiences and compelling counter-arguments;

(3) their content is impossible;

and he emphasizes that

(4) underlying all delusional *judgements* is a transformed *experience* of reality.

Jaspers goes on to describe in detail three subgroups of delusions proper: delusional perception, delusional idea or notion, and delusional awareness.

In *delusional perception* there is an immediately experienced change of meaning of a particular perception, though the perception itself remains unaltered. The basic feature is the 'establishment of an unfounded reference' (Gruhle 1915). A popular example (Arthur 1964) is of a man who looked at the marble tables in a café and suddenly became convinced that the end of the world was coming. It is important, as is claimed in this instance, that the tables are correctly perceived and appreciated and that the content of the delusion is incomprehensibly related to the patient's life and situation.

Schneider's original (1959) claim that it was possible to identify delusional perceptions by form alone, with no reference to content, is convincingly refuted by Spitzer (1990), who gives an example. In order to distinguish between a normal person who saw a black cat crossing her path on a Friday the 13th and thought it meant bad luck, and a schizophrenic patient who saw a black dog crossing his way and thought it meant the end of the world, criteria of 'understanding' and 'cultural background' have to be applied. 'Delusional perceptions are neither unmistakable in form nor can one ignore their content' (Spitzer 1990, p. 385). Spitzer instead suggests that because delusional perceptions are linked to some observable object they are more easily detected and less ambiguous than other delusional phenomena, and are therefore to be rated higher on a continuum of detection than other delusional items. 'What we have in mind is not a clear-cut dichotomy, but rather a continuum, on which delusions may be placed, ranging from "very questionable, might be just ingenious, or might be just a religious phantasy" to "certainly delusional".' (Spitzer 1990, p. 386).

Jaspers' sudden *delusional ideas* appear as sudden notions, new aspects and new meanings of remembered life experiences. Jaspers quotes a patient who wrote to him:

It suddenly occurred to me one night, quite naturally, self-evidently but insistently, that Miss L. was probably the cause of all the terrible things through which I had to go these last few years . . . if you examine it fairly you will see there is very little reflection about it; rather everything thrust itself upon me, suddenly, and totally unexpectedly, though quite naturally. I felt as if scales had fallen from my eyes and I saw why life had been precisely as it was . . . . (Jaspers 1913, p. 103)

Delusional awareness (Wahnstimmung) is characterized by a knowledge of immense and universal happenings without clear ideation or sensory perception. Merely thinking about things gives them a special significance, for they seem to be linked, in some way, with so many other things.

Central to Jaspers' concept of delusion is incorrigibility. Decisive in characterizing this is not the subjective intensity of the experience but the maintaining of what is evident to the patient in the face of subsequent reflection and external criticism. Jaspers accepts that any individual may assert a truth against the beliefs of the majority, but for the deluded person the incorrigibility serves a particular interest: 'The delusional content is of vital necessity . . . and without it he would inwardly collapse. . . . In the case of delusion, we may see someone irretrievably lost in untruth.' (Jaspers 1913, p. 411).

Jaspers regards primary delusions as deriving from an alteration in the personality, the precise nature of which is unknown, or from a hypothetical disease process, and while the pre-morbid personality might explain the content or theme of the delusion it cannot explain the actual existence of a delusion. Thus, as Schmidt (1940) points out, if it were always possible to derive a primary delusion from one of the closely related primary symptoms with which it is intimately associated, or from some underlying disorder, then it would no longer be a primary but a secondary delusion, and there would be no such thing as a genuine delusion.

Spitzer (1992) suggests that Jaspers' interest in dividing delusions into primary and secondary is best understood within the context of psychiatric knowledge at his time. The spirochete which causes syphilis had just been discovered and Jaspers expected that the pathogenic agent causing Kraepelin's dementia praecox (Kraepelin 1899) would sooner or later be found. Meanwhile the diagnosis of such a disease process had to be based on psychopathology. The distinction between the understandable development of delusions (such as in mood disorders) and the non-understandable delusions caused by a supposed disease process was therefore of great importance.

Matussek (1952) has, however, argued that Jaspers' approach of distinguishing between the 'psychological irreducibility' of some delusions and the understandable nature of others has had serious implications. It implies that the former phenomena can only be explained in organic terms, and discourages attempts to investigate their psychological structure regardless of cause.

Winters and Neale (1983) note that the distinction between primary and secondary delusions is less popular in German-speaking countries than it has been in Britain and the United States. They argue that the distinction is neither reliable, nor of any proven diagnostic significance, despite Schneider's (1959) claim that delusional perception is of exceptional diagnostic importance to schizophrenia.

Delusional perception nonetheless remains an intriguing sub-type of delusion (or a point along the continuum) and it is possible that such delusions involve subtle alterations in perceptual qualities, such as vividness, in contrast to the grosser perceptual changes found in hallucinations.

Spitzer (1990) also considers in detail Jaspers' three defining characteristics. The third characteristic, impossibility (or falsity) presents a number of problems, which are discussed below (pp. 5–6). Spitzer, however, notes that if one concentrates on falsity, one is likely to overlook the remaining two characteristics, subjective certainty and incorrigibility. These, he argues, when about the subject's own mental states, are typical of normal people. 'Statements like "I'm feeling pain" . . . or "I'm thinking at the moment" can be uttered by me with subjective certainty and incorrigibility and there is no way in which somebody could ever reasonably question these statements' (Spitzer 1990, p. 390). Spitzer thus proposes, modifying Jaspers, that a delusion can be said to be present only when these two characteristics occur in beliefs about the *external* world, and *not* when the belief concerns the person's own mental states.

Modern definitions

Definitions of delusions, as well as the primary/secondary distinction, reflect, in British and North American psychiatry, the profound influence of Jaspers, and standard definitions incorporate many of the characteristics of delusions that he described. Mullen offers the following definition in a textbook of psychiatry:

A delusion is an abnormal belief. Delusions arise from disturbed judgments in which the experience of reality becomes a source of new and false meanings. Delusions usually have attributed to them the following characteristics:
(i) They are held with absolute conviction.
(ii) They are experienced as self-evident truths usually of great personal significance.
(iii) They are not amenable to reason or modifiable by experience.
(iv) Their content is often fantastic or at best inherently unlikely.
(v) The beliefs are not shared by those of a common social or cultural background. (Mullen 1979, p. 36)

Such a definition presents a number of difficulties. There is evidence (for example Strauss 1969) that many delusions do not show absolute conviction. Furthermore, psychiatric texts do not specify how 'absolute' conviction is to be assessed, whether by obtaining a simple statement of certainty or by a more rigorous test of the precise level of conviction. Secondly, while delusions are said to be 'not amenable to reason' (or incorrigible), criteria are again not laid down for assessing this: should the interviewer present compelling counter-arguments, and, in such a context, what counts as 'compelling'? The assessment of the fantastic or bizarre nature of the content presents problems. A number of researchers have failed to achieve satisfactory inter-rater reliability only on ratings of bizarreness (Kendler *et al.* 1983; Flaum *et al.* 1991; Junginger *et al.* 1992).

Moor and Tucker (1979) discuss problems with the criteria of falsity and deviance of delusional beliefs. They argue that false beliefs are common, and if having a false belief were a sufficient condition for having a delusion, then many, if not most, people would be delusional. The occurrence of false beliefs, particularly unusual ones, may, they suggest, be taken as a sign of a delusion, but it should not be regarded as a defining condition. The problem with the criterion of deviance is the difficulty of choosing the 'right' group as the reference class. They note that a distressing consequence of accepting the deviant belief view is that it helps to legitimize the use of psychiatric treatment for political repression against minorities with dissenting opinions.

More recently Walkup (1990) has argued that some delusional beliefs are not so much false as *unfalsifiable*, because, like certain religious beliefs, they do not make truth claims, that is factual claims about states of affairs in the world. He proposes that these unfalsifiable delusions are essentially descriptions of subjective experience, although this may not always be immediately obvious. As an example, Walkup gives 'I didn't do that' referring to a patient's arm movement, witnessed by observers. However, the patient, he argues, may in fact be (correctly) describing his experience of the arm movement as alien.

Spitzer (1990) would, however, argue that Walkup's classification of 'unfalsifiable delusions' are not in fact delusions but rather 'disorders of experience', since delusions are, by his account, statements about *external reality*. We will be returning to the relationship of belief to experience in subsequent chapters.

Spitzer (1990) also cites other difficulties with the criterion of falsity. He suggests that some delusional statements, while they do make truth claims, are unfalsifiable in practice, for example the claim that the patient is being followed by the CIA. Additionally, it has long been recognized that certain delusions may be true, whether coincidentally or as a consequence of the delusion itself: delusions of jealousy may fall into this category.

Mullen (1979), in discussing his definition, asserts that the conditions of absolute conviction and imperviousness do not serve alone to distinguish deluions from normal beliefs and common error. He emphasizes the idiosyncratic nature of the belief's content when compared with the beliefs of those common to the individual's social group (i.e. he espouses the deviant belief view). Mullen's concept of the delusion's origin is Jasperian: it is 'to be sought in some as yet little understood disruption and change of mental function which fundamentally alters the patient's knowledge of the world' (Mullen 1979, p. 36). Mullen, in common with other writers, notes that a true belief may coincidentally be a delusion; thus the way that the belief emerges and the reasons for its acceptance will determine whether it is classified as a delusion. He also accepts the Jasperian distinction between primary and secondary delusions, in terms of the criterion of being understandable. The primary delusion is 'an ultimately irreducible phenomena [*sic*] not amenable to psychological understanding and only explicable finally in terms of the causal connections governing the presumed organic changes in the brain' (Mullen 1979, p. 38). Mullen ends his discussion with a statement which, like Jaspers', reflects a view of an unassailable dichotomy between delusions and normal beliefs: 'Delusion represents a profound and complex disorganisation of mental life stretching way beyond mere false ideas and mistaken beliefs' (Mullen 1979, p. 40).

Definitions in diagnostic systems, for example the *Diagnostic and statistical manual* (DSM III-R) (American Psychiatric Association (APA) 1987), also assume a dichotomy between delusions and normal beliefs. The DSM III-R definition states:

Delusion. A false personal belief based on incorrect inference about external reality and firmly sustained in spite of what almost everyone else believes and in spite of what constitutes incontrovertible and obvious proof or evidence to the contrary. The belief is not one ordinarily accepted by other members of the person's subculture (i.e. it is not an article of religious faith).

The Present State Examination (Wing *et al.* 1974), unlike the DSM III-R, allows for full delusions and 'partial delusions', which, while definitely present, are expressed with doubt, and also preserves the tradition of a primary/secondary distinction.

Dichotomy or dimension?

The notion of a simple presence/absence of a delusion has been questioned for some years. Despite the absolutist language of much that Jaspers wrote, he himself raised the question of whether the delusion is to be comprehended 'as a break in the normal life-curve or simply as part of the continuum of personality development' (Jaspers 1913, p. 98). In 1968, Strauss published an influential paper in which he argued that delusions (and hallucinations) are not discrete and discontinuous, and that they may be better (and more accurately) conceptualized as points on a continuous distribution from the normal to the pathological. He reported that interviews with 119 patients yielded about one-half as many questionable delusions as definite ones (142 '?' and 269 positive) even when using the Present State Examination (PSE) categorization, which allows for partial delusions. He proposed that symptoms should be described and rated in terms of the extent of deviation from normal functioning along a variety of dimensions. Spitzer (1990) also has suggested that delusions may lie along a continuum.

The difficulty in achieving a clear definition perhaps lies in a naivety about the way in which language is used to define concepts. Wittgenstein (1953) challenged the idea that the concept 'game' could be defined simply:

Look for example at board games, with their multifarious relationships. Now pass to card games; here you find many correspondences with the first group, but many common features drop out, and others appear. When we pass next to ball games, much that is common is retained, but much is lost. Are they all 'amusing'? Compare chess with noughts and crosses. Or is there always winning and losing, or competition between players? Think of patience. In ball games, there is winning and losing; but when a child throws a ball at the wall and catches it again, this feature has disappeared . . . and the result of this examination is: we see a complicated network of similarities overlapping and criss-crossing: sometimes overall similarities, sometimes similarities of detail.

I can think of no better expression to characterise these similarities than 'family resemblances'; for the various resemblances between members of a family: build, features, colour of eyes, gait, temperament, etc. etc. overlap and criss-cross in the same way. — And I shall say: 'games' form a family. (Propositions 66–67)

Fulford notes that Wittgenstein introduced a method of conceptual analysis which, rather than proposing a priori definitions of terms, is based upon 'careful, comprehensive observations of linguistic data (including the ways in which and the purposes for which concepts are actually employed in any given real-life situation . . .)' (Fulford 1989, p. 22). Applying such an analysis to delusions, Fulford also notes that 'notwithstanding the wide acceptance of the conventional definition, not all delusions show all or even any of these features' (Fulford 1989, p. 202).

In a recent chapter an approach compatible with Wittgenstein's is advanced which offers a possible partial resolution to the difficulty (Oltmanns 1988). Oltmanns suggests that a definition of delusion should incorporate a list of defining characteristics, none of which is necessary or sufficient:

a. The balance of evidence for and against the belief is such that other people consider it completely incredible.
b. The belief is not shared by others.
c. The belief is held with firm conviction. The person's statements or behaviours are unresponsive to the presentation of evidence contrary to the belief.
d. The person is preoccupied with (emotionally committed to) the belief and finds it difficult to avoid thinking or talking about it.

e. The belief involves personal reference, rather than unconventional religious, scientific or political conviction.

f. The belief is a source of subjective distress or interferes with the person's occupational or social functioning.

g. The person does not report subjective efforts to resist the belief (in contrast to patients with obsessional ideas).

Any given belief may possess one or more of the features. Beliefs that clearly exhibit all of these features will undoubtedly be considered delusional. As some of the features are omitted or become less obvious, there will be less agreement about the classification of the belief. Oltmanns also suggests that some of the features may be more important, for predicting treatment response or with regard to particular aetiological mechanisms, and that this is a matter for empirical investigation.

The definitions of Jaspers and of Oltmanns differ in two important respects. Firstly, there is a shift from Jaspers' view of delusions as clearly present/absent, to beliefs being considered 'more or less delusional' (Oltmanns 1988, p. 5), and secondly the number of defining characteristics has grown, from three to seven. Delusions are more complex phenomena, it is argued, than Jaspers acknowledged. There are two other crucial changes, in underlying assumptions: Jaspers saw the primary/secondary distinction as central, and primary delusions as essentially irrational; Oltmanns makes no such distinction, and avoids any conclusion about the rationality of the deluded subject's unresponsiveness to contradictory evidence. It would, however, be a mistake to assume that Oltmanns' views are generally accepted. Most psychiatric practice, in Britain and North America, continues to be influenced by Jaspers, and to treat delusions as dichotomous with normal beliefs, either primary or secondary, and as fundamentally irrational.

IRRATIONALITY

For Jaspers, the deluded person is 'irretrievably lost in untruth', incorrigible despite subsequent reflection and external criticism. For Mullen (1979), 'delusions arise from disturbed judgments' which are not amenable to reason. The DSM III-R regards delusions as based on *incorrect inference* about external reality. These present a view of delusions (and their holders) as irrational. It is not, however, clear in what respect they are irrational, and it is hinted that the failure of reasoning is two-stage: in their formation and, perhaps more strikingly, in their subsequent maintenance. In the next chapter the model of rationality that these views embody will be considered, and alternatives discussed; it is sufficient to note here that irrationality is typically assumed to be characteristic of or responsible for delusions.

OCCURRENCE OF DELUSIONS IN 'SCHIZOPHRENIA' AND OTHER DISORDERS

Delusions are present in a wide variety of conditions. Manschreck (1979) and Maher and Ross (1984) have pointed to more than 75 clilnical conditions that are accompanied by delusions. These include psychiatric, neurological, metabolic, and endocrine disorders. They are regarded as marker symptoms for the presence of a psychotic disorder, and in particular are central to the diagnosis of schizophrenia (Cutting 1985).

Some delusions, particularly Jasperian 'primary' delusions, and beliefs about control of body, will, mind, or mood and about thought interference, are said to be characteristic of schizophrenia, while other types of delusion, paranoid or of reference, are more common in this group, but occur in all psychotic conditions (Cutting 1985). Yet others, Cutting argues, — grandiose, poverty, guilt, bodily change, disease — also occur in schizophrenia but are more characteristic of affective psychosis.

Winters and Neale (1983) note that formal thought disorder rather than delusions was considered, for many years, to be pathognomonic of schizophrenia. As a result, psychological research focused heavily on studies of formal thought disorder. However, delusions are more common than formal thought disorder in psychotic patients. They quote data from the International Pilot Study of Schizophrenia (IPSS; World Health Organization 1973) which found, among 306 project-consensus schizophrenics representing nine different countries, delusions of reference in 67 per cent, delusions of persecution in 64 per cent, and delusions of control in 48 per cent. Formal thought disorder occurred in only about 10 per cent of the sample. Winters and Neale also note a modest association between type of delusion and diagnosis, in the IPSS data. While many delusions were not predictive of diagnosis, two types were moderately predictive. Of the 27 patients with delusions of control, 96 per cent were diagnosed as suffering from schizophrenia or paranoid psychosis, and of the 227 patients with delusions of grandiosity, 92 per cent were given a diagnosis of manic psychosis.

To restrict a study of delusions to those that occur in 'schizophrenia' would clearly limit unduly the domain of interest; at the least, comparisons between diagnostic groups may yield new findings. The relative importance of specific symptoms for schizophrenia continues to be problematic, as does reliably distinguishing between certain diagnostic categories, particularly between schizophrenia and the affective disorders (Kendell and Brockington 1980; Cutting 1985; Bentall *et al.* 1988).

Persons (1986) has argued for the study of particular symptoms such as delusions, hallucinations, and thought disorder, rather than of syndromes. She argues that there are six important advantages to the single-symptom approach:

(1) avoidance of misclassification of subjects;

(2) the study of important phenomena which are often ignored;

(3) facilitation of theoretical development;

(4) isolation of single elements of pathology for study;

(5) recognition of the continuity of clinical phenomena with normal phenomena; and

(6) improvements in diagnostic classification.

In the present work, it is therefore assumed that delusions merit study in their own right, and that such a study (although not the focus here) may also ultimately assist further clarification of the diagnostic debate. However, in that delusions are said to be pathognomonic of schizophrenia, and of no other condition, much that has been previously written about delusions, refers to those of schizophrenics, and so work relating to schizophrenia will necessarily take a prominent place.

TYPES OF DELUSION

Content classifications

The most common method of categorizing delusions is by content (Maher 1988), and numerous lists can be found in psychiatric textbooks, the rarer content-types perhaps sporting the French name of their discoverer, such as 'De Clérambault's' (the delusion of believing falsely that one is loved, or erotomania), or an esoteric term derived from Greek, such as 'lycanthropy' (delusion of becoming a wild beast).

Bleuler (1911, trans. 1950) in his classic work on *Dementia praecox or the group of schizophrenias* lists delusions classified by content.

Wing *et al.* (1974) in the Present State Examination provide a categorization which combines categories created atheoretically simply from an inspection of content, for example fantastic delusions, delusions of pregnancy, and others with an implicit theoretical basis, for example primary delusions, or delusions of control (referring to Schneiderian first-rank symptoms of schizophrenia).

Others have grouped delusions with a similar content, according to a (sometimes implicit) theory of their origin. Thus the DSM III (American Psychiatric Association 1980), in its list of eight types, includes a category of 'mood-congruent' delusions. Cutting (1987), in comparing the content of delusions in patients with a diagnosis of schizophrenia and those with acute organic psychosis, used a content classification suggested by Cummings (1985): simple persecutory, complex persecutory, hypomanic (mood-congruent), and associated with neurological deficits.

Finally, there are studies of groups of delusions, chosen for their similar content, for example those with a theme of misidentification (Christodoulou 1986).

Classification by hypothesized aetiology

Some categorizations are not determined by content, but by association with other symptoms, or by the formal structure of the delusion. Clearly Jaspers' (1913) work is of this type. Two early French psychiatrists, Dupré and Logre (1911), classify on the basis of the hypothesized aetiology of the delusion. They categorize three types of delusional states: hallucinatory delusional states, misinterpretative delusional states, and confabulatory delusional states. In the first, it is argued, the predominant disorder is of perception; in the second, the disorder is assumed to derive from errors of logic, perception being unaffected; in confabulatory states the subjects' ideas do not arise from false perceptions or false reasoning but from a 'fiction of endogenous origin, a subjective creation. Misinterpretation is a cognitive process, confabulation a poetic process.' (Dupré and Logre 1911, p. 161).

Syntactic structure

Maher (1988) argues that the classification of delusions on the basis of their content has been relatively unfruitful, in terms of identifying associations with differing aetiology, prognosis, and treatment response. He is unimpressed with claims that such classification systems predict diagnosis, since criteria for diagnosis typically include reference to the class of delusion. Maher proposes instead that belief systems, including delusions, can be classified along epistemological lines, such as empirical—falsifiable or hermeneutic—interpretative.

Heilbrun and Heilbrun (1977), in an investigation of a theory of delusion formation in process and reactive schizophrenics, conducted a content analysis of delusions based chiefly on grammatical and semantic aspects of transcripts of deluded subjects' speech. A number of process-reactive differences emerged, in, for example, the extensiveness (total number of clause units), the variation of content, and the inductive—deductive reasoning (as assessed by the ratio of positive to negative subjective state verbs).

To conclude, while current psychiatric classification systems emphasize content categories on the basis of a superficial analysis of content, or linked to presumed diagnostic types, earlier (Continental) psychiatrists proposed categories on the basis of theories of delusion formation. This approach has been echoed in the more recent work of psychopathologists, who have suggested categorizing delusions in terms of their formal structure, rather than surface content.

ON DISTINGUISHING DELUSIONS FROM OBSESSIONS AND HALLUCINATIONS

Although, up to this point, we have been concerned with what, if anything, distinguishes a delusion from a 'normal' belief, there can also be a difficulty in drawing a clear distinction between delusions and other abnormal thoughts, notably obsessions. Mayer-Gross *et al.* (1969) described an obsession as 'a mental event with a subjective sense of compulsion over-riding an internal resistance', but added that if the personality as a whole identifies itself with the idea, then it may be considered as a delusional idea. Mullen (1979) also noted that the resistance to an obsession may fluctuate and suggested that in such cases the phenomenon would only be called a delusion if the lack of resistance becomes not an occasional but a constant feature of the experience.

Oltmanns makes reference to this difficulty, by including among his criteria for delusion a distinction from obsession: '(g) The person does not report subjective efforts to resist the belief (in contrast to patients with obsessional ideas).' (Oltmanns 1988, p. 5). This is not entirely satisfactory. There is considerable evidence that not all obsessionals resist their ideas (for example Stern and Cobb 1978), without losing their characteristic obsessionality, that is psychiatric consensus would continue to regard certain such phenomena as un-equivocally obsessional. Moreover there is no clear evidence that certain delusions are *not* resisted; empirical studies of this are absent. Turning to Oltmanns' criteria for delusions (see pp. 8–9 for the full list), few would dispute that (d) to (f) are common in obsessions, (g) is sometimes present, and, it can be argued, (a) to (c) are not uncommon.

As beliefs, obsessions, and delusions may share characteristics common to all beliefs (for example intensity of conviction), or to a subcategory of 'abnormal' beliefs (for example dysfunctional sub-jective distress); however, if it is possible for an obsession to share all the features of delusions (as listed by Oltmanns) clearly a definitional problem exists.

One approach to this problem may be to consider the formal properties of the phenomena, in particular the logical structure as some have argued (above) for classifying delusions. While most, if not all, delusions are expressed as finished and established truths, obsessions, on the other hand, even when expressed with firm and intense conviction, do often appear as conditional propositions: a doubt that, a fear that, a belief that unless . . . . They are also typically accompanied by preventive, corrective, or neutralizing acts to stave off the feared outcome. At times, in some obsessionals, the conditional mode of thinking becomes overshadowed by a propositional mode: the disaster *has* occurred (or definitely will, regardless). Thus one possible method for distinguishing between the phenomena may be to classify on the basis of predominant logical mood. A study would be required to test this proposal.

Another psychiatric symptom from which delusions must be distinguished is the hallucination. Conventionally, there is no prob-lem here: whereas a delusion is a belief, a hallucination is a perception. Thus, while the two phenomena may be closely linked, for example a patient may have a delusional belief about the source of some 'voices', the judgement and the experience can be clearly distinguished. There are, however, some problems. We have already noted that some delusions are said to be descriptions of disordered experience, such as delusions of control, or thought broadcasting. A fundamental problem is posed by distinguishing between perception and judgement. There is evidence, which we will address in Chapter 3, that pre-existing beliefs can influence (even determine) experience (Slade and Bentall 1988) so that someone who expects to hear a tune played may report actually hearing it, even though it is not played. The relationship between hallucinations and delusions will be further addressed in subsequent chapters.

ACCESSING (OR ASSESSING) DELUSIONS

In the foregoing discussion, an important problem has not been addressed: how can we know about delusions? Delusions as beliefs are essentially private phenomena, subjective states of the mind. Most students of delusions simply ask the person thought to be deluded to tell them what they believe, and infer from the verbal behaviour (the statement) to the internal state. There are obvious difficulties with this. The person may lie, or otherwise deliberately attempt to mislead. The person may misunderstand what is being asked, or be operating from a culturally different frame of reference. The person may be distracted and give an inaccurate response. The person may wish to please the questioner, or to bring the interrogation to an end, and answer accordingly. All these are problems which by no means are restricted to the study of delusions, but apply also to the study of a variety of internal processes (for example mood states); they are not in themselves reasons for not asking the questions, but rather for asking them with due care, and regarding the responses with due caution.

A further difficulty, also relevant to other phenomena, but which may particularly apply to this category of disturbed (in some sense) thinking, is the Nisbett and Wilson (1977) problem of 'telling more than we know'. In a study of normal subjects' accounts of reaching a decision, they found that subjects constructed plausible accounts of their mental processes, rather than accessing the actual process. Much of this construction process is rapid and not accessible to consciousness. It may be that when asking people with delusions to give an account of their delusions, especially of the *process* of, for example, acquisition, we may be likewise asking them to tell more than they can know.

DELUSIONS AS BELIEFS

An important concern here is whether delusions are best described as beliefs. A number of theorists have disputed this. Spitzer (1990) has suggested that they are 'knowledge claims', rather than beliefs, since beliefs, by his account are not expressed with conviction and certainty. Fulford (1989) has argued that some delusions are not false beliefs, but value judgements (about, for example, the subject's unworthiness).

Berrios (1991) has made the stronger claim that no delusions are beliefs, in that they do not fulfil certain philosophical criteria for beliefs (Price 1934) largely because deluded people typically fail to consider alternative hypotheses. He therefore proposes that delusions be regarded as 'empty speech acts'.

However, Berrios is here basing his argument on a formalized philosophical construct of belief, rather than on naturalistic studies of belief claims. In the next chapter we will consider a number of psychological studies of belief formation and change which demonstrate that normals do not always fulfil formal criteria; thus if delusions are not (ever) beliefs, nor are many phenomena conventionally regarded as such.

For the present, therefore, we will treat delusions as generally describable as beliefs while acknowledging the views that some may be value judgements, some statements of subjective experience, and some knowledge claims.

DELUSIONS AND BEHAVIOUR

One approach taken by some to the problem of assessment is to study other aspects of the subject's behaviour, thought to be associated with the internal belief state (Paul and Lentz 1977). However, the relationship between belief and behaviour is complex and no simple inference can be made from the latter to the former (Wessely *et al.* 1993). In the case of delusions, it has been suggested that the extent to which they direct actions is extremely variable (for example Mullen 1979). The behaviour of the deluded person is therefore of interest, but cannot be studied as a substitute for the attempt to assess more directly the subjective experience of belief. A fuller understanding of the subjective experience, moreover, should assist with the study of associated actions, as a recent paper demonstrates (Buchanan *et al.* 1993). The focus of this book, however, is on delusional beliefs, and not on the behaviour of people with delusions.

CONCLUSIONS

The concept of delusion has been dominated, in Anglo-American psychiatry, by the thinking of Jaspers (1913). However, while the primary/secondary distinction remains embedded in much current thinking, recent definitions do not emphasize this distinction, nor do they list Jaspers' primary delusions, delusional perception, delusional idea, and delusional awareness. There is a shift from Jasperian views to a more atheoretical descriptive approach. Modern psychiatric definitions continue, however, to present operational and conceptual problems, such as determining when a delusion is false, bizarre, incorrigible, or subculturally deviant, or distinguishing delusions from obsessions. There is a separate problem, which we will return to later, of the relationship between belief and experience, a question which has ramifications for our understanding of hallucinations. We prefer a dimensional view in which delusions are, following Strauss (1969), not viewed as discrete and discontinuous with normal beliefs, but as sharing characteristics with the latter, so that for any given dimension (belief strength, preoccupation, systematization, etc.), a delusion may be placed at any point along the continuum. Many delusions will, it is predicted, lie at extreme points on some, but not all, identified continua. A list of defining characteristics of the type given by Oltmanns (1988) reflects therefore more accurately than earlier, less complex definitions, the phenomenon of delusion.

We accept that the Oltmanns' approach does not solve all the conceptual problems which have been raised, and in particular the status of delusion as 'belief' poses important questions; however, for the present we will continue to view delusions within this framework while acknowledging that it has limitations. Unlike some recent critics, however (for example Harper 1992), we do not view delusion as a concept no longer likely to yield interesting findings, but rather see the resurgence of interest in the phenomenon as potentially productive.

Although delusions are said to be particularly characteristic of schizophrenia, and much that is written about delusions is in the context of discussion of schizophrenia, it is proposed here that the study of delusions should not be limited to those found in subjects bearing such a diagnosis. The validity of the construct of schizophrenia is in some doubt (Bentall *et al.* 1988; Boyle 1990), and the wide variety of conditions in which delusions occur, and the need to consider them in detail, point to the usefulness of studying delusions in their own right, independent of diagnostic categorization.

The classification of delusions has been hitherto influenced by surface content, and to a lesser extent, association with diagnosis. Maher (1988) has argued that these methods have not proved fruitful, and proposes considering the formal (grammatical) structure of delusional belief statements. The value of such an approach warrants empirical investigation, and may help with the problem of distinguishing obsessions from delusions.

An important theme in the literature on delusions is their irrationality. For many, the hallmark of delusion, is incorrigibility, being 'not amenable to *reason*'. It is this issue of rationality and reason which will be considered next.

2 Reasoning, rationality, and delusions

INTRODUCTION

Incorrigibility is one of Jaspers' central criteria for identifying delusions, characterized by the maintaining of what is evident to the patient in the face of subsequent reflection and external criticism. This feature is retained in some form in all subsequent descriptions or definitions, so that delusions are said to be:

(1) 'firmly sustained in spite of what almost everyone else believes and in spite of what constitutes incontrovertible or obvious proof or evidence to the contrary' (DSM III-R, American Psychiatric Association 1987);

(2) 'not amenable to reason or modifiable by experience' (Mullen 1979);

(3) 'unresponsive to the presentation of evidence contrary to the belief' (Oltmanns 1988; see Oltmanns and Maher 1988);

(4) 'maintained unshakably in the face of reason' (Freedman *et al.* 1975).

In addition to incorrigibility, some definitions make explicit reference to judgemental processes. While some assert that the reasoning of the deluded individual may remain intact, (for example 'it is not a disturbance of intelligent grasp . . . the disturbance is one of symbolic meaning' (Mayer-Gross *et al.* 1969, p. 272)), other definitions impute a fault in the judgemental processing (for example 'pathologically falsified judgments' (Jaspers 1913); 'a false personal belief based on *incorrect inference* about external reality' (DSM III-R) [our emphasis].

Theories of the formation and maintenance of delusion are discussed in Chapter 6; here it is proposed to consider models of rationality and of normal reasoning in order to clarify the concepts of incorrigibility and faulty judgement in delusions.

THEORIES OF REASONING AND RATIONALITY

A theory of knowledge, incorporating a norm of rationality, is implicit in most definitions of delusions: they argue that individuals should (and if normal do) reformulate their beliefs when presented with 'incontrovertible' evidence to the contrary. Reed makes this view explicit:

Delusions are notoriously unshakeable. Whatever counter-evidence is presented, however much experience denies it, the delusion remains firm. No amount of persuasion, argument and demonstration can serve to convince the deluded patient of the falsity or irrationality of his belief. Normal beliefs, however cherished, can be changed or modified by education, persuasion, coercion or the cumulative effect of contradictory evidence. (Reed 1988, p. 143)

Some philosophers have argued that human beings possess an innate mental logic and that it is against logical norms that the performance of individuals should be assessed (see Johnson-Laird (1982) for a full discussion). The evidence is at odds with this view. Frequent deviations from logical standards such as those imposed by the laws of syllogisms are to be found, even in logically sophisticated human beings (for example Chapman and Chapman, 1959; Wason and Johnson-Laird 1972; Dickstein 1978).

Others have, in contrast, proposed theories of deductive reasoning that render people inherently irrational (for example Erickson 1974; Evans 1980; cited in Johnson-Laird 1982). By these accounts, even if an individual draws a conclusion that happens to be valid, the underlying thought process fails to be logical since the theories preclude a complete examination of the consequences of the premises.

Such views, Johnson-Laird continues, inflate the importance of logic. A valid deduction is one which follows necessarily from the premises: if the premises are true, then the conclusion must be true. But it is entirely possible to argue validly from false premises. Moreover, any set of premises yields an infinite set of valid conclusions, most of which are wholly trivial, such as a conjunction of all the premises. Hence, when drawing a specific valid conclusion, one must be guided by more than logic. Other principles must be applied to avoid trivial conclusions.

Johnson-Laird summarizes the debate about human reasoning:

Some theorists, principally philosophers, argue that we are invariably rational; other theorists, principally psychologists, argue that we are invariably irrational. But these contrary points of view are not exhaustive.

There remains a third possibility . . . human beings may well be rational in some circumstances, but not in others. (Johnson-Laird 1982, p. 3)

One philosophical account of empirical reason is the method of simple induction, in which knowledge is acquired by the accumulation of observations of instances: thus a person can know that the sun will rise tomorrow, because it has always risen every day (Russell 1912). Clearly, despite the fact that there may have been innumerable instances of the truth of an event, and none of its falsehood, it is possible that this will not be true in the future, as in the famous example 'All swans are white', refuted by the discovery of black swans.

Philosophers of science, in attempting to describe the acquisition of scientific 'knowledge', have rejected the simple empiricist position that beliefs are essentially descriptions or generalizations concerning experience. Popper (1959) proposed a theory of falsificationism: that scientific knowledge is/should be advanced by positing hypotheses which are to be tested, and, where possible, refuted. Knowledge is not so much advanced by the accumulation of correct ideas, as by the rejection of false ones.

However, Kuhn (1962) criticized Popper's approach as being inaccurate historically, and untenable philosophically, and proposed instead that in periods of 'normal science' a group of scientists sharing a research field make, and should make, advances *not* by refutation, but by a tenacious process of confirmation of a shared paradigm.

W.V.O. Quine, a logician, had in the early 1950s already proposed a theory consistent with Kuhn's position:

Total science is like a field of force whose boundary conditions are experience. A conflict with experience at the periphery occasions readjustments in the interior of the field. Truth values have to be redistributed over some of our statements . . . But the total field is so under-determined by its boundary conditions, experience, that there is much latitude of choice as to what statements to re-evaluate in the light of any single contrary experience . . . . If this view is right, it is misleading to speak of the empirical content of an individual statement — especially if it is a statement at all remote from the experiential periphery of the field . . . Any statement can be held true come what may, if we make drastic enough adjustments elsewhere in the system. Even a statement very close to the periphery can be held true in the face of recalcitrant experience by pleading hallucination or by amending certain statements of the kind called logical laws. (Quine 1953, pp. 42–3)

Lakatos (1970) also, while disputing some points with Kuhn, accepts the view that no single experimental result can ever kill a theory, since any theory can be saved from counter-instances either by some auxiliary hypotheses or by a suitable reinterpretation of its terms. All scientific research programmes are characterized by a 'hard core' of hypotheses; research activity is not directed at this core but at the auxiliary hypotheses which form a protective belt around the core. This is the negative heuristic of the programme: the result of a methodological decision to cordon off the core of a theory from the threat of refutation. The hard core, within Lakatos' framework, is only rejected when the programme ceases to predict novel facts and there is available a rival research project which explains the previous success of its rival, and also supercedes it by a further display of heuristic power.

Scientists, Lakatos argues, are not irrational when they ignore counter-examples: no research programme will predict all possible outcomes, and thus 'refutations' must be expected. Thus, scientists frequently disregard apparent counter-evidence in the expectation that later work will convert it to empirical support, provided the work is theoretically progressive (Gholson and Barker 1985).

Philosophers of science, therefore, allow for 'rational' incorrigibility under certain conditions. Experimental studies in the psychology of inference also demonstrate that a simple falsificationism is absent under certain conditions in normals.

EXPERIMENTAL STUDIES OF REASONING IN NORMALS

Confirmation bias

A large number of studies have demonstrated a phenomenon dubbed 'confirmation bias' (see Wason and Johnson-Laird 1972; Einhorn and Hogarth 1978; Ross and Anderson 1982), a tendency to perceive more support for prior beliefs than actually exists in the evidence at hand.

In one experiment, in which subjects were required to construct a hypothesis, Wason and Johnson-Laird found that subjects approached the task with a verification method, ignoring alternatives and only seeking to confirm the chosen hypothesis. In this context, perhaps most noteworthy is the theory holder's response to equivocal or ambiguous data. As Lord *et al.* (1979) have documented, potentially confirmatory evidence is apt to be taken at face value while potentially disconfirmatory evidence is subjected to highly critical and sceptical scrutiny. Individuals in such circumstances are apparently acting very like the scientists of Kuhn (1962) and Lakatos (1970).

Wason and Johnson-Laird further comment how, in certain of their reasoning experiments, subjects became convinced of the correctness of their theories: 'When a subject has succeeded in arriving at a generalisation which has been supported by confirmatory evidence, he [*sic*] seems to exert a proprietary right over it — it is his own creation' (Wason and Johnson-Laird 1972, p. 240). Some even demonstrated what the researchers considered to be behaviour characteristic of deluded individuals, although in no sense were these people 'ill', and although they returned to 'normal' after the task. The subject's attention is funnelled on the first decision and 'he contradicts himself . . . and denies the facts which confront him' (Wason and Johnson-Laird 1972, p. 239). This occurred when the material was abstract rather than concrete, as if such material is too arbitrary and tenuous to manipulate mentally; it provides no intrinsic check for errors and no reassuring contact with reality.

Belief in the paranormal

A particularly relevant area of research in normal psychology is research into belief in the paranormal. French (1992) has recently written an interesting review of this literature. He reports, firstly, that belief in paranormal phenomena is widespread in the normal population and, secondly, that evidence suggests that cognitive biases in information processing underlie such beliefs. Thus he quotes a poll of 1236 adult Americans (Gallup and Newport 1991) which found that one in four believe in ghosts, one in four believe they have had telepathic experiences, one in ten claim to have seen or been in the presence of a ghost, one in ten claim to have talked to the devil, and one in seven say they have personally seen an unidentified flying object (UFO). French reports on a number of studies which have investigated information processing in those who believe in the paranormal compared with those who do not. These have shown the former to exhibit reasoning bias, including confirmation bias, poor appreciation of the probability of coincidences, and other systematic errors.

Over-confidence

Over-confidence in judgements has also been studied experimentally. Meehl's (1954) classic book on clinical prediction demonstrated that people's impressions of how they reason, and how well they reason, could not be taken at face value. Lichtenstein *et al.* note that in matters of general knowledge of moderate or extreme difficulty, over-confidence is a 'pervasive' finding (Lichtenstein *et al.* 1982, p. 314). In a study by Fischhoff *et al.* (1977) of judgements of factual questions, extreme over-confidence is demonstrated. For example, on one task subjects expressed 100 per cent certainty on responses that were four times out of five incorrect. Fischhoff *et al.* note how uncritical of their inferences many subjects are, quoting another researcher, Johnson-Abercrombie:

The[se erroneous] inferences were not arrived at as a series of logical steps but swiftly and almost unconsciously. The validity of the inferences was usually not inquired into; indeed the process was usually accompanied by a feeling of certainty of being right. (Johnson-Abercrombie 1960, p. 89)

Kahneman and Tversky (1973) used the term 'the illusion of validity' to describe people's confidence in highly fallible judgements. Einhorn and Hogarth (1978) consider why this illusion persists, and why experience fails to teach people to doubt their fallible judgement. They propose a cognitive, rather than a motivational account for this, and highlight the practical and theoretical difficulties that individuals have, in the 'natural environment', in making use of disconfirming information.

In a task in which a judgement is made for the purpose of deciding between alternative courses of action, the outcome information, which is available when actions are taken, may be the only source of feedback on judgement. Einhorn and Hogarth consider the hypothetical case of a manager learning about his or her predictive ability concerning the potential of job candidates. Suppose the manager follows a rule, 'my judgement is highly predictive'. The crucial factor here is that actions are contingent on judgement. Therefore, at a subsequent date, the manager can only examine successful candidates to see how many are successful. If there are many successes, these instances all confirm the rule. Einhorn and Hogarth argue that in such circumstances it would be difficult to disconfirm the rule, even though it might be erroneous. Thus large amounts of positive feedback can lead to reinforcement of an invalid rule and hence to the 'illusion of validity'. This work emphasizes that the evidence which is taken into account is crucial in making an inference.

In addition to the difficulty of learning from disconfirming information, Einhorn and Hogarth argue that the coding in memory of outcomes as frequencies rather than probabilities (Estes 1976) has major implications for explaining the persistence of the illusion of validity. Estes showed that subjects made predictions on the basis of the number of positive occurrences (frequencies) rather than that number, divided by the total possible instances (probabilities). They suggest that one reason for this may be the confirmation bias, in which subjects fail to pay attention to the non-occurrence of the event of interest. In these studies, a relationship thus emerges between the confirmation bias and over-confidence.

Belief perseverance (or incorrigibility)

Biases at the stage of the *formation* of an inference are matched by similar biases concerned with *maintaining* beliefs, once formed. Ross and Anderson (1982) describe a number of studies which demonstrate belief perseverance both in the face of new data and after evidential discrediting. In a fascinating study, Lord *et al.* (1979) first selected subjects who either supported or opposed capital punishment as an effective deterrent. The subjects were then presented, in a counter-balanced design, with two purportedly authentic empirical studies. One seemingly provided empirical support for their position and the other seemingly opposed it. At strategic points in the reading of these two studies, the two groups completed ratings on the quality of the studies and their own beliefs. Both proponents and opponents of capital punishment consistently rated the study that supported their beliefs as 'more convincing' and 'better conducted' than the study that opposed those beliefs. Also, the net effect of reading both studies was to polarize still further the beliefs of the groups.

Ross and Anderson (1982) conclude that there can be little doubt that our beliefs influence the process by which we seek out, store, and interpret relevant information. Indeed, such processes make manageable the innumerable items of information with which each person is presented at every moment. They posit a number of mechanisms underlying these phenomena, including biased search for and interpretation of the evidence, and a tendency to search for causal explanations which, once found, tend to buttress and sustain the original belief, even in the face of subsequent challenges. In a concluding paragraph, one important point is mentioned: beliefs do change. Apart from change in the face of massive amounts of disconfirming evidence, or decisive well controlled experiments, the authors suggest that vivid, concrete, first-hand experience may be effective under certain (as yet unspecified) conditions in bringing about belief change.

Alloy and Tabachnik (1984) and Alloy (1988) consider the effect of the strength of the prior belief and the strength of 'current situational information' on the likelihood of belief change. They argue that when an individual has a strongly held prior theory, new information will be less effective in changing the theory than that same information when the prior belief is weakly held. They also propose that when strong expectations and strong current evidence are in conflict, the individual is faced with a cognitive dilemma, and is more likely to favour the expectations, overlooking or distorting the current information. The Lord *et al.* (1979) study quoted above is consistent with this view. These papers call to mind Lakatos' relatively irrefutable 'hard core', and the auxiliary hypotheses at which a critical appraisal may be directed. A final point, emphasized by Alloy (1988), addresses the question of expectation change: according to the model, situational information not only combines with pre-existing expectations to influence judgements, but also modifies the very expectations with which it interacts. In this regard the model is dynamic and does not preclude change.

Experimental paradigms relevant to the integration of new data with pre-existing expectations

It is apparent that judgements concerning the relationship between events (including those that are internally generated) are influenced by pre-existing expectations, which, in part, are dependent on previously observed regularity. Two paradigms derived from animal learning theory, and recently applied to human subjects, illustrate this clearly. The Latent Inhibition Paradigm (LI) (Lubow *et al.* 1982), is presented in Table 2.1. It consists of two stages, pre-exposure and test. In the first stage, a stimulus is repeatedly presented to the organism (PE); in the second stage the pre-exposed stimulus is paired with reinforcement in any of the standard learning procedures, classical or instrumental. When the amount of learning is measured, relative to a group that did not receive the first stage of stimulus pre-exposure (NPE), it is found that the pre-exposed group learn the association much more slowly. In the version of the test developed for use with human subjects, during the pre-exposure phase subjects are

Table 2.1 *Latent Inhibition paradigm*

		Test
Pre-exposure (PE) group	A–A——A–A	A–X
No pre-exposure group (NPE)	——	A–X

In normals, pre-exposure to A reduces rate of learning the A–X association. This is usually interpreted as reflecting a reduction in the deployment of attention to a redundant stimulus.

either pre-exposed to a to-be-conditioned stimulus (white noise) or not pre-exposed; during the test phase, measurement is made of the speed with which all subjects learn an association between this stimulus and the addition of points to a scoreboard. A masking task is provided by asking all subjects to count occurrences of nonsense syllables during the pre-exposure phase (Baruch *et al.* 1988). The effect of pre-exposure is considered to indicate a reduction in the deployment of attention to a predictable, redundant stimulus. The 'regularity' operating to influence expectations is that the stimulus has no consequences.

A second paradigm, Kamin's (1969) blocking effect, possesses many of the same features as LI and is illustrated in Table 2.2. Again it involves a pre-exposure phase in which the experimental group learns an association between two stimuli (A−X); control subjects learn either no association or a different one at this stage. Following this both groups are presented with pairings between a compound stimulus (A + B) and X. Both groups are then tested for what they have learnt about the B−X relationship. The pre-exposed group demonstrates less learning than controls; this is the 'blocking' effect, and it is generally agreed to result from a process in which attention to B is reduced because it is found to predict nothing in addition to what is predicted by A (Pearce and Hall 1980). In the test developed by Jones *et al.* (1992) for use with human subjects the blocking task was in the form of a computer game in which subjects were presented with a series of differently coloured shapes and required to predict when a yellow square would appear. For pre-exposed subjects the yellow square was always preceded by a blue square. For control subjects yellow triangles were randomly preceded by triangles of other colours. Procedure was then identical for both groups in the two following stages. In stage 2, the yellow square was always preceded by a compound of a blue square and a computer-generated tone. In

Table 2.2 *Blocking paradigm*

	Phase 1	Phase 2	Test
Blocking group	A−X	(A + B) − X	B−X
Control group	——	(A + B) − X	B−X

In normals, the control group learns B−X faster than the blocked group. This is usually interpreted as reflecting reduction in attention to B in phase 2 for the blocked group, because it is found to predict nothing additional to that predicted by A, that is it is redundant.

stage 3, the yellow square was always preceded by a tone. The blocking effect was evident in poorer learning to this tone in stage 3 in the pre-exposed group.

A later version of the 'blocking' test developed by Jones (personal communication) employs as stimuli the names of 'film stars', the outcome being the success or failure of films in which they appeared, either singly or jointly. Again, a clear 'blocking' effect has been demonstrated. It is apparent that on this task we are moving close to the attribution of a causal role to the 'film star' stimuli. White (personal communication) suggests that 'at some point the record of experiences (and other information) becomes a causal belief such as "X has the power to produce Y" or "X is a possible cause of Y"'. It will be argued in our final chapters that not only is an abnormal view of the relationship between events a prominent feature of delusional thinking, but also that at times this proceeds to the perception and/or attribution of abnormal causal relationships.

Causal processing in normals

From the immediately preceding discussion it is clear that the normal processes of *causal* perception, inference and attribution, are therefore relevant to our enquiry. As White has pointed out, 'Philosophers are concerned with what causation actually is . . . psychology is concerned with how people understand and perceive causation, make causal attributions and so forth' (White 1990, p. 10). However, he notes that philosophical theories can serve as models for psychological theories, and experiments may be carried out to determine the extent to which people's behaviour conforms to such philosophical theories. Hence psychologists within different research traditions have focused on specific aspects of causality emphasized by different philosophers.

Einhorn and Hogarth (1986) have argued that the assessment of cause is best viewed as a judgemental process occurring under conditions of uncertainty. Causal reasoning is considered to take place in order to make sense of the world, and is more likely to happen when events violate expectations and are seen as unusual. Temporal order, and spatial and temporal contiguity, are clearly crucial to a judgement of causality. Thus Shanks *et al.* (1989), employing a computer game, have demonstrated that increasing delays between an action and an outcome lead to progressively lower judgements of causality. When temporal or spatial contiguity is low, inferring causality becomes more difficult, and requires the use of intermediate causal models to bridge the spatial and temporal gap.

Einhorn and Hogarth (1986) also attach great importance to the cue of 'covariation' consistent with traditional notions of cause put forward by Hume (1739/1964) and Mill (1872). It is suggested that these cues, contiguity and covariation, together with similarity of cause and effect (for example congruity of duration and magnitude), may be combined to predict the gross strength of a perceived causal relationship. The constraints operating in the construction of an extended causal chain are considered to be those involved in a single causal link, namely temporal order, contiguity, congruity, and covariation. However, a further factor is important, the 'schema' or 'theory' that people bring to bear in a particular situation. This may be either acquired by experience or innate. Nisbett and Ross (1980) have argued that prior conceptions of causal relationships may outweigh considerations of mere data-driven estimates and result in such phenomena as 'illusory correlations' (cf. Chapman 1967). The important role played by a consideration of specific alternative explanations has also frequently been emphasized. We therefore begin to see clear links between research on causal reasoning and that on probabilistic inference described above. Both concern how subjects update their present beliefs on the basis of new information.

Covariation is regarded as informative about causation since it is believed that the world is sufficiently stable for a given causal mechanism to operate in the same way from one occasion to the other. Indeed, in science one is attempting 'to explain types of occurrence that usually or normally happen' (White 1990, p. 9). However, in commonsense one is frequently attempting to explain a particular event that is a departure from what is normal. White argues that Einhorn and Hogarth's (1986) analysis is inappropriate to many instances of causal reasoning, and that 'people will only use covariation information when an event has passed some initial test of plausibility as a potential cause of the effect in question' (White 1989, p. 435). In suggesting this he draws upon Harre and Madden's (1975) concept of the 'powerful particular', an object or person with a certain type of property, namely the power to produce certain sorts of effects. White suggests that in many instances causal relationships can be directly perceived, and that 'much if not most causal processing is automatic' (White 1989, p. 437).

Here 'automatic' is being employed in the sense introduced by Shiffrin and Schneider (1977). Their theory attempted to integrate work in the related areas of selective attention, visual search, and short-term memory search. Automatic processes are seen as involving the activation of a fixed sequence of mental operations in response to a particular input configuration. They involve direct access to long-term memory, require no processing capacity, and occur outside of conscious awareness. Extensive training results in the development of automatic processing, but once established it is relatively inflexible and difficult to suppress. In contrast, controlled processes are temporary sequences of mental operations under the control of the individual. They require attention, involve demands on limited processing capacity and are often serial in nature. Although relatively slow, and subject to interference by other simultaneous controlled processing, they can be flexibly adapted to task requirements. Thus, a highly skilled and experienced typist will perform the task of typing with automatic processing, whereas a person learning to type will require attention to stimuli and responses, that is will operate on controlled processing. White argues that Einhorn and Hogarth's (1986) model is describing causal reasoning using controlled processing.

It is thus suggested by White that causal processing is frequently part of the automatic processes involved in perception and that 'it does not require attentive deliberation, and it is constructive, interpretative or inferential to no greater or lesser extent than perception in general' (White 1989, p. 438). It makes use of familiarity with the causal powers of a variety of objects and events. White draws upon developmental research to argue that causal processing begins by being automatic, and that controlled causal processing is a later development, being brought into operation only when automatic processing cannot be employed.

White (1989) suggests that controlled causal processing does not occur on every occasion that automatic processing does not. Certain information will not be subject to any causal inference. Controlled causal inferences and attribution of the kind described by such as Kelley (1973) are considered to occur when they promote the practical interests and concerns of the person making the attribution. Controlled causal processing is therefore more open to influence by individual needs and preoccupations. Although such judgements are frequently inaccurate with respect to the principles of inference and analysis considered 'normative' by scientists, they may not be so when judged against an individual's current practical concerns. Beliefs about causal relationships may on occasions be tested before being accepted, but the evidence is suggestive of a strategy of positive instance testing rather than a search for covariation information. This is clearly similar to the more general reasoning biases which have been well documented, and which have been discussed above.

CONCLUSIONS

At the beginning of this chapter it was noted that delusions have been viewed as irrational, because of their characteristic incorrigibility and an unspecified faulty judgement. It is clear, however, that belief perseverance is not abnormal, nor even always undesirable, whether the field of enquiry is science or everyday life; 'rational' incorrigibility may occur under certain conditions. Both ordinary people and professional scientists may be justified in favouring their expectations in the face of incongruous information; nevertheless, this bias may also lead to errors.

Experimental psychology and philosophy are seen to describe over-confidence in judgements, a bias to confirming rather than refuting beliefs, the perseverance of beliefs in the face of contradictory information, and causal inferences which may be 'automatic' or, when 'controlled', inaccurate by normative standards. 'People systematically violate principles of rational decision-making when judging probabilities, making predictions or otherwise attempting to cope with probabilistic tasks' (Slovic *et al.* 1977). While at times a motivational account may be offered for these behaviours, re-searchers such as Ross and Anderson (1982) argue that cognitive or 'informational' processes also operate, such as ignoring the informa-tional value of non-occurrences. There has been debate over the extent to which the documented shortcomings in human judgement are as pervasive as suggested by some theoreticians (Kihlstrom and Hoyt 1988); however, it is now uncontroversial that 'human judgement and inference are not always logical and rational, and that certain types of errors creep into the process' (Kihlstrom and Hoyt 1988, p. 90).

These findings, and others which demonstrate 'deviations' in the inferential performance of normals from 'rational' behaviour (as defined by, for example, formal models of logic) has led psycho-logists to consider the rules by which individuals do form and maintain judgements, with resultant new models, both normative and descriptive, for understanding human inferential performance. These models include Bayesian models of probabilistic inference (Fischhoff and Beyth-Marom 1983), reasoning with mental models (Johnson-Laird 1983), and the specification of judgement heuristics (guiding principles) which individuals employ in different inferential tasks (for example Tversky and Kahneman 1982).

Finally, it is important to note that the biases documented above, assumed to arise, at least in part, from the limited processing capacity of memory, are not unvarying. They differ both with the context of the task and the type of information to be stored (for example Johnson-Laird 1982; Lichtenstein and Fischhoff 1977).

It thus appears that delusional incorrigibility is less abnormal (or irrational) than the definitions imply. It is possible that the phenomenon represents a quantitative rather than a qualitative difference from normal performance or, intriguingly, that maintaining an already strongly held belief in the face of contradictory evidence is not, in itself, at all abnormal. Possibly the *formation* rather than the maintenance of a delusion is, in some way, biased. It is possible to use these psychological models to investigate and specify such biases if found. Theories of delusional belief formation and maintenance are discussed in full in Chapter 6; we consider next studies in the reasoning processes of psychotic patients.

3 Studies of reasoning in people with psychosis

INTRODUCTION

While there have been numerous studies of a variety of aspects of information processing in psychotic (normally defined as 'schizophrenic') subjects, the frequency of published papers concerning reasoning in subjects specifically identified as *deluded* is considerably lower. The specific studies of deluded subjects will be discussed first, and the more general work then considered briefly.

REASONING IN PEOPLE WITH DELUSIONS

Von Domarus (1944) proposed that delusions arose from a failure of syllogistic reasoning. This failure rests on an inability to distinguish between the identity of subjects and the identity of predicates in logical propositions. According to the Von Domarus principle, a patient might reason thus:

> Napoleon was exiled and incarcerated
> I am incarcerated
> Therefore I am Napoleon.

Experimental studies have not provided support for this proposition. Two studies are reported which attempted to test the theory. Nims (1959, quoted in Williams 1964) compared 25 hospitalized male schizophrenics with 25 normal controls and found no significant differences on overall performance of logical reasoning. However, the precise fallacy, of the similarity of the predicates specified by Von Domarus, was not examined.

Williams (1964) compared 50 hospitalized normal patients and 50 schizophrenics controlled for education and IQ on three types of syllogism, including the type specified by Von Domarus, and with varying content (personal, impersonal, abstract, and concrete). He found no significant differences between the groups (who both made a large number of errors) on the experimental items. However, Williams comments in the discussion of the findings that 'each or most' of the schizophrenic subjects may have 'recovered temporarily from the psychotic episode and were functioning normally with regard to intellectual functions at the time of testing' (Williams 1964, p. 58). It appears that there was no requirement that the subjects were currently psychotic, and none that they were (or ever had been) deluded. Such an admission considerably weakens the study as a test of Von Domarus' theory.

A series of studies did, however, employ deluded subjects, investigating not their logical reasoning but their response to ambiguous perceptual stimuli. McReynolds *et al.* (1964) proposed a conceptualization of delusions as attempts to 'make sense' of the environment, reducing intolerable inner tensions at the expense of distortion of reality. It was hypothesized that the tendency to form delusions constitutes a generalized adaptive pattern in which ambiguous stimuli are more likely to be organized into 'meaningful wholes'. They compared 24 delusional and 25 non-delusional schizophrenics on a test which involved deciding what is represented in incomplete pictures of common objects. The deluded subjects attempted more pictures and identified more pictures correctly than the nondeluded group.

Abroms *et al.* (1966) followed up the study of McReynolds *et al.* by again presenting ambiguous images, but they grouped their subjects by severity of paranoid ideation and of delusions. They found that the paranoid subjects were more likely to make inaccurate judgements than suspend judgement when presented with ambiguous stimuli. The tendency was more pronounced with increasing severity of 'paranoid trait'.

Delusional paranoid schizophrenics were compared with non-delusional paranoid schizophrenics and alcoholic controls by McCormick and Broekema (1978) on a perceptual recognition task. The paranoid patients, in contrast to the other two groups, rarely showed sequential learning, but almost exclusively employed a 'jump to conclusions' response strategy, expressing 100 per cent certainty of their correctness on the basis of one response, responding 'suddenly and impulsively'. Both schizophrenic groups showed over-confidence about their ratings of ambiguous slides. The authors conclude that the paranoid (deluded) subjects 'respond to each stimulus as if it is new, neither integrating information from earlier slides to facilitate that performance nor showing the debilitating effects of earlier incorrect responding' (McCormick and Broekema 1978, p. 396).

In the 20 years following the mid-1960s, with rare exceptions (such as McCormick and Broekema), experimental work in the inference of deluded subjects seems largely to have ground to a halt, perhaps because the syndrome of schizophrenia was successfully competing for researchers' attention (Persons 1986).

The 1980s have witnessed a resurgence of interest in the inferences of deluded subjects. In 1984, Brennan and Hemsley compared paranoid and non-paranoid schizophrenics on their formation of 'illusory correlations' (Chapman 1967); the paranoid subjects, selected by the Maine Scale (Magaro *et al.* 1981) were deluded while the non-paranoids exhibited thought disorder, incongruity of affect and hallucinations. An illusory correlation is the report by an observer of a correlation between two events which in reality are not correlated, or not to the extent reported. Brennan and Hemsley found that the paranoid group reported particularly strong illusory correlations, compared with non-paranoid and normal groups, on a task involving stimuli relevant to subjects with paranoid delusions.

In a study of inference in subjects specifically selected for the presence of persecutory delusions (Kaney and Bentall 1989), attributional style was investigated. Social attribution theory (Kelley 1967) provides a framework for understanding the explanations that individuals give for their own behaviour and the behaviour of others. Kaney and Bentall argue that this perspective is appropriate, since many of the delusions experienced by psychotic patients seem to concern the patient's place in the social universe and his or her beliefs about the intentions of others. The deluded subjects were compared with matched depressed controls and normal controls. Like the depressed subjects, the deluded patients made excessively global and stable attributions for significant events. However, in contrast to the depressed subjects, the deluded subjects made excessively external attributions for negatively valued events and excessively internal attributions for positively valued events.

A difference was also found on scores on the Magical Ideation Scale (Eckblad and Chapman 1983), a scale which measures superstitious ideas and beliefs in magical phenomena, the deluded subjects scoring more highly than either control group. Kaney and Bentall (1989) suggest that this may simply reflect the deluded subjects' tendency to make external attributions for unwelcome experiences. An alternative considered is that deluded patients tend falsely to detect covariation between randomly associated events, that is to see coincidences as significant. Such a disposition to perceive causal relationships inaccurately might, they argue, plausibly be a source of vulnerability to delusions and is consistent with the findings of Brennan and Hemsley (1984).

Bentall *et al.* (1991) extended the investigation of social attributions in deluded subjects. Employing the same subjects (with one exception) as Kaney and Bentall (1989), they studied the choice of person, circumstance, and stimulus attributions in a paper-and-pencil task giving social vignettes describing interactions between two persons (not including themselves). Thus, for a given interaction subjects are asked to attribute the cause of the event to the actor (person), to the context in which the action occurred (circumstance), or to the target of the action (stimulus). Subjects were also asked to rate how certain they were in their choice, on a five-point scale, ranging from very certain to very uncertain. It was found that the deluded patients made excessive person attributions for negative events. They were also excessively certain about their judgements, compared with the depressed controls. Just as the deluded subjects in the Kaney and Bentall (1989) study were unwilling to attribute negative events of which they were the victim to themselves, so in this study they were unwilling to blame the victim in negatively valued social interactions in which they were not involved. Bentall *et al.* thus argue that this bias in the social reasoning of deluded subjects has a protective function, which would also explain the subjects' unwillingness to countenance the possibility of being mistaken.

The above studies offer a basis for forming hypotheses about the reasoning of deluded subjects.

A number of studies suggest that deluded subjects may exhibit a tendency to 'jump' to perceptions when presented with ambiguous perceptual stimuli. Over-confidence, particularly on the basis of single items of information, may also be characteristic. In a recent review of this work, Butler and Braff (1991) comment that this characteristic judgemental style may be associated with the formation and maintenance of delusions.

Brennan and Hemsley (1984) suggested that there may be a content-specific bias in detecting covariance among paranoid subjects and the studies of Bentall and Kaney and colleagues have found attribution biases for social situations and excessive certainty among deluded subjects about their judgements. These studies employed material concerning social and interpersonal situations, situations which may not be neutral with respect to the subjects' abnormal beliefs; reasoning on a 'content-neutral' task in deluded subjects has not been investigated.

REASONING IN SCHIZOPHRENIC SUBJECTS

There have been a very large number of studies concerned with aspects of thinking (attention, perception, learning, and inference) in schizophrenia which clearly bear some relation to reasoning and judgement in deluded patients. However, much research in schizophrenia takes no account of the current (or past) delusional status of subjects. A person can receive a DSM III diagnosis of paranoid schizophrenia in the absence of delusions if she or he has hallucinations with persecutory or grandiose content (Persons 1986). Therefore, only a brief summary will be given of this work.

Fleminger (personal communication), in a discussion of delusional misidentification syndromes, summarized studies on the processing of perceptions and memories in patients described as having schizophrenia. He argues that three main conclusions can be drawn:

1. Such patients make early perceptual hypotheses when faced with ambiguity (McReynolds *et al*. 1964; Abroms *et al*. 1966; McCormick and Broekema 1978), which may or may not lead to errors. They jump to perceptions.

2. There is a disruption of the effects of context and expectancy. Weakening of the effects of context is sometimes observed (Levy and Maxwell 1968; Hemsley 1987), although patients with 'paranoia' may be more easily influenced by contextual cues than those with 'schizophrenia' or non-psychotic psychiatric controls (Ross and Magaro 1976).

3. There are difficulties in responding to the gestalt qualities of the scene, and they concentrate instead on detail (Matussek 1952; Schwartz Place and Gilmore 1980; Cutting 1985). This results in difficulties in the perception of faces and of facial expression.

It should be noted, although Fleminger does not comment on this, that all the studies cited in support of this first point, jumping to perceptions, as we have noted above, compared deluded with non-deluded subjects, and find this phenomenom more commonly in the former group.

His second conclusion, the weakening of the effects of context and expectations, is more generally thought to apply to 'schizophrenics' in contrast to those diagnosed as 'paranoid'. Magaro strongly espouses this view:

Paranoids rely on a rigid conceptual process without adequate constraint from perceptual data — stimulus features stripped of conceptual loading —

while schizophrenics rely primarily on perceptual data without adequate categorisation and classification from conceptual processes. (Magaro 1984, p. 191)

Hemsley (1987) has proposed that 'weakening of the influence of stored memories of regularities of previous input on current perception' occurs in schizophrenia. Thus schizophrenics are less able to make use of the redundancy and patterning of sensory input to reduce information processing demands.

A number of studies provide support for Hemsley's hypothesis. The study of illusory correlations (Brennan and Hemsley 1984), reported above, found that whereas the paranoid group made strong illusory correlations on tasks which involved stimuli relevant to paranoid delusions, the non-paranoid group produced weaker illusory correlations (that is, more accurate performance) than normals. The 'schizophrenics' were not imposing a pattern on the data, while the 'paranoid' subjects did so excessively.

Baruch *et al.* (1988) compared acute and chronic schizophrenics and normals on a task measuring latent inhibition, the retardation of learning that normally occurs when a subject forms an association to a stimulus previously repeatedly presented without consequence (discussed in Chapter 2). The acute subjects demonstrated disrupted latent inhibition, that is they failed to make use of the prior learning, and thus learned the new association more quickly. Chronic medicated schizophrenics did not show this effect, and the performance of the acute group normalized following six to seven weeks of medication.

Jones *et al.* (1992) report similar findings for acute schizophrenics when the 'blocking' paradigm is employed. In this group there was no effect of pre-exposure to the A–X contingency (cf. Table 2.2). Indeed they learned the B–X association significantly faster in the pre-exposure condition. Thus, both studies indicate an alteration in the way current information is integrated with previously presented material.

Two major contrasting styles of information processing are thus identified in the literature on schizophrenia: some patients appear to 'concentrate on detail at the expense of theme' (Cutting 1985), ignore past learned regularities, and respond to the stimulus immediately present. Others (often described as paranoid) impose meaning on current experience employing strong prior expectations.

One possibility is that this second style represents an adaptive strategy of 'simplified' cognitive structuring of experience. For a normal subject, the expectancies generated will be sensitive to subtle variations in context. If this process is disturbed, the initial response could be a reduction in the number of categories employed. The proposal is reminiscent of Radley's (1974) suggestion that 'paranoid schizophrenics may maintain a relatively "simple" or tight system of constructs in the face of invalidation, by forming idiosyncratic and univalent impressions of others' (cf. Chapter 6). We will return to this issue in the final chapter.

HALLUCINATIONS AND REASONING

Some research has been conducted on inferences made by hallucinating subjects. Certain delusions are thought to arise out of attempts to explain abnormal perceptual experiences (a theory which will be fully discussed in Chapter 6); whether or not this is so, many deluded subjects also report hallucinations, and thus the inferential processes involved in the hallucinatory experience are of interest.

Barber and Calverley (1964) found that if instructed to close their eyes and listen to the record 'White Christmas', about 5 per cent of their (normal) subjects would subsequently report believing that the record had been played. This work led Mintz and Alpert (1972) to consider whether the ability to imagine vivid auditory stimuli is a necessary, although not sufficient, condition for hallucinations and whether hallucinators are as aware as non-hallucinators of the distortions they introduce into their perceptions of verbal stimuli. Using the 'White Christmas' test with hallucinating schizophrenics, non-hallucinating schizophrenics, and normal controls, they found that hallucinators were more likely than controls to report hearing the record (75 per cent) and to believe that it had been played (10 per cent). They propose a model of hallucination formation in which vividness of auditory imagery and defective reality testing are necessary but not sufficient factors.

Slade and Bentall (1988), in a comprehensive review of the research into the cognitive mechanisms of hallucinations, identify a central process: making a distinction between imagined events (experiences generated by the subject) and events in the external world. This process, 'reality testing' or 'reality discrimination', has long been studied in normals, and Slade and Bentall argue that the evidence suggests that inferential processes are implicated in this skill.

Recent work in the field comes from Johnson and Raye (1981), who have studied the process of distinguishing between memories of events and memories of thoughts. They have identified a number of cues that people use to make this distinction, for example the greater the effort at recall, the more likely the product will be considered self-generated (Johnson *et al.* 1981). Slade and Bentall argue that hallucinations result from a dramatic failure of the skill of reality discrimination, leading the hallucinating individual to misattribute repeatedly his or her self-generated events to an external source. Thus the 'error might not lie in the information that is available *but in the inferences that the person makes on the basis of that information*' (authors' italics; Slade and Bentall 1988, pp. 214–15). They quote a number of studies consistent with this hypothesis, including a reinterpretation of Mintz and Alpert (1972) as demonstrating not imagery vividness but a reality discrimination failure, and conclude: hallucinators make over-rapid perceptual judgments and are more willing than non-hallucinators to believe that a perceived event is real. It is not surprising, therefore, that they tend to mistake their own cognitive processes . . . for events in the external world (Slade and Bentall 1988, p. 220).

This view is in marked contrast to a view implicit in much psychiatric writing on hallucination (for example DSM III-R, (APA 1987)) in which the phenomenon is construed as a given abnormal percept.

CONCLUSIONS

The literature on the reasoning of deluded people is sparse. Some early studies suggested no abnormalities, but were methodologically and conceptually flawed. Other work indicates that some inferential biases may operate, at least with ambiguous perceptual, delusion-relevant, or social and interpersonal material. Inferences concerning neutral material have not been extensively studied.

The studies conducted with schizophrenic patients, despite the conceptual and methodological difficulties discussed, do again appear to indicate some biases in processing data. This work and the work on hallucinators suggests that some patients make rapid and over-confident judgements about their perceptual experiences, are less influenced by previous learned associations, concentrate on detail not theme, and show impaired reality discrimination.

It is therefore of interest to study further inferences in deluded subjects, not in a spirit of demonstrating their irrationality, but to seek to identify characteristic inferential biases, if any, which may contribute to the formation or maintenance of their delusional beliefs. Studies of reasoning in deluded subjects will be reported in Chapters 7 and 8.

4 The assessment of delusions*

INTRODUCTION

There are clearly a number of approaches to the assessment of delusions, including the analysis of the unstructured speech of a deluded person, structured self-report and observer ratings made on the basis of structured interviews. The purposes of assessments are also variable: for example, to assist in diagnosis, to assess global treatment outcome, to investigate the 'structure' of delusions and to assess change in delusions.

A concept of delusion, even if not explicit, is always embodied in these different approaches, and more recent methods reflect the shift from viewing delusions as all-or-nothing phenomena to conceptualizing them as beliefs deviating to a greater or lesser extent from normal beliefs along a number of dimensions. This multidimensional view is, however, not universal and psychiatric assessment devices still tend towards unidimensional approaches, even where a simple dichotomous (presence/absence) framework has been abandoned (Garety 1992a). Standard definitions (as we have noted above, Chapter 1) also propose that delusions are fixed, immutable, and impervious to counter-evidence. In this chapter a new method for assessing dimensions of delusions is presented, together with new assessments of the responsiveness of delusions to disconfirming evidence.

Different types of assessments of delusions can be found embedded in a wide variety of other assessment devices, such as diagnostic interviews like the Present State Examination (Wing et al. 1974), global symptom assessments (examples include the Comprehensive Psychopathological Rating Scale (Asberg et al. 1978) and the Brief Psychiatric Rating Scale (Overall and Gorham 1962)), and instruments designed to record 'positive' symptoms such as the Scale for

* The content of this chapter incorporates shortened and revised versions of two previously published papers: Garety, P.A. (1985). Delusions: problems in definition and measurement. *Br. J. Med. Psychol.*, **58**, 25–34 and Brett Jones, J., Garety, P.A., and Hemsley, D. (1987). Measuring delusional experiences: a method and its application. *Br. J. Clin. Psychol.*, **26**, 257–65.

the Assessment of Positive Symptoms (Andreasen 1984). A review of these and other scales can be found in Garety (1992*a*) and Garety and Wessely (1993).

INSTRUMENTS FOR ASSESSING DELUSIONS

A small number of instruments have been designed specifically to assess delusions. These range from extensive interviews to individual questions designed to assess a particular aspect of delusional experience.

The Personal Ideation Inventory (Rattenbury *et al.* 1984; Harrow *et al.* 1988) is a semi-structured interview designed for use in research, to further knowledge about delusions by an investigation of 'three major dimensions of delusional ideation'. It consists of 71 items covering premorbid concerns, conviction, commitment, and perspective. 'Commitment' refers to the immediacy of the belief or how impelling and important it feels to the patient, and draws on cognitive signs, such as preoccupation, and behavioural signs, such as influence on daily activities. 'Perspective' refers to the patient's view as to whether others will regard the ideas as strange or implausible. The scale is observer-rated, in that the interviewer assigns scores to the subject's responses, based on predetermined categories.

The Maudsley Assessment of Delusions Schedule (MADS) (Buchanan *et al.* 1993; Taylor *et al.* 1993) is also an observer-rated research instrument for the elicitation of the detailed phenomenology of a delusion. It draws on work described in this book and thus provides for a multidimensional assessment. Eight dimensions are assessed: conviction, belief maintenance, affect, action, idiosyncrasy, preoccupation, systematization, and insight. The action subscale is fairly lengthy and is a useful starting point for the assessment of behaviour associated with delusions. This interview has good inter-rater reliability and is reasonably sensitive to change, although not suitable for frequent repeated testing.

Kendler *et al.* (1983) administered a semi-structured interview in which ratings were made by the interviewer of conviction, extension, bizarreness, disorganization, and pressure. Adequate, if not high, inter-rater reliabilities were achieved for most of the dimensions. The sensitivity of the interview to change was not investigated.

In Chapter 5, another instrument, the Characteristics of Delusions Rating Scale (Garety and Hemsley 1987) will be described. This is a visual analogue scale, designed to assess 11 self-rated aspects of delusional experience.

The instruments described above suffer from some limitations for the clinician and researcher interested in the treatment of delusions. As lengthy and wide-ranging schedules they are generally not suitable for the repeated detailed assessment of targeted change. To overcome this limitation a new assessment method was devised. It draws on an existing methodology, the Personal Questionnaire technique, and was designed to provide a reliable measure, which is also sensitive to small changes, of any chosen dimension of a delusion. Secondly, with the exception of the MADS, which incorporates modifications of the work described here, the instruments also do not address systematically the role of evidence and experience in the formation and maintenance of the delusion. Further assessments, designed to address this, are also described.

PERSONAL QUESTIONNAIRE TECHNIQUES FOR ASSESSING DELUSIONS

The Personal Questionnaire (PQ) approach was developed by Shapiro (1961). He was interested in producing a reliable, individual-centred method which could be used to scale changes in subjective reports about symptoms during the course of psychological treatments. Shapiro's PQ was therefore developed primarily as a practical clinical tool.

The measure described here is a modification of Shapiro's original PQ, the Ordinal Personal Questionnaire (Phillips 1977). The technique provides ordinal scaling of successive levels of symptoms by means of statements representing different levels of symptom intensity. It has been used for a wide variety of symptom statements, but, except in the very early stages of construction of the method (Shapiro and Ravenette 1959), it has not been used to scale aspects of delusions.

A PQ consists of two stages, a construction stage and a stage of administration and scoring. The first stage involves a careful interview with the patient in order to ascertain the psychological symptoms of which he or she complains; in the case of delusions these may involve statements of conviction, or distress or preoccupation. Following this, a number of variants of the original statements are chosen, each one reflecting a different level of symptom intensity. The original statement, and the variants, are specific to the individual subject and use the subject's own wording, although suggestions may be made by the interviewer. The statements are then written on separate index cards. At this stage it is important that the interviewer checks that the subject scales the set of statements consistently, with statements thought to represent a higher level of symptom intensity placed above those thought to represent a lower level. If this is not done, the statements are reworded until the subject is able to use them consistently. The second stage involves a series of occasions on each of which judgements of symptom intensity at that time are obtained.

The PQ method is therefore a particularly suitable approach to use for assessing delusions. It can be tailored precisely to the individual and uses his/her own linguistic and conceptual framework. This is particularly helpful with suspicious or paranoid subjects. It is sensitive to change and has built-in methods for checking both the scaling and reliability of responses to individual items (Phillips 1970). It is also simple to construct and score. The first study of the use of PQs with deluded subjects explored the measurement of the intensity of conviction (Garety 1985). The fixity, or incorrigibility, of the belief is also measured if administration is repeated with, where desired, intervening presentation of counter-evidence. Personal Questionnaire techniques have also subsequently been employed to assess delusional preoccupation (Brett-Jones *et al.* 1987) and mood disturbance associated with a delusion (Chadwick and Lowe 1990).

In this chapter we will describe the first application of the PQ technique to assess delusional intensity and fixity.

METHOD

Two subjects were selected for this first study. No attempt was made to modify the subjects' beliefs for the period of the trial: the aim was simply to explore the feasibility of reliably measuring the intensity and fixity of given sets of beliefs over time, and the sensitivity of the measure to change.

The first subject (PJ) was a 33-year-old patient with a long-standing diagnosis of paranoid schizophrenia. Although on relatively high doses of phenothiazines, he frequently and spontaneously uttered paranoid statements, agreed unequivocally by clinicians involved in his care to be delusional, for example 'the birds are blaming me', 'dogs avoid me', and 'people call me dangerous when they see me'. His delusions were regarded as chronic, fixed, and untreatable.

The second subject (RF) was a 39-year-old man who had recently been admitted to hospital, after approaching Buckingham Palace claiming to be 'the Queen's son'. He had no previous psychiatric history, and was provisionally diagnosed as suffering from a 'schizo-phreniform psychosis'. He had been unwilling to come into hospital and was therefore compulsorily detained under Section 2 (later Section 3) of the 1983 Mental Health Act, on the grounds of his delusions. He commenced phenothiazine medication by week 2 of the trial.

Administration

The first stage of construction of the PQ involved eliciting 'de-lusional' statements from the subjects, and agreeing the wording for the expression of differing levels of intensity of beliefs, for example 'dogs avoid me' was expressed in five statements:

Form (i): That dogs avoid me is — definitely true
                        "   probably true
                        "   may be true or false
                        "   probably false
                        "   definitely false.

An alternative scaling of the same belief concerning dogs was also considered:

Form (ii): I know that   — dogs avoid me
          I believe very stongly that —   "
          I believe that   —   "
          I have a few doubts that   —   "
          I doubt that   — dogs avoid me.

It was considered that form (ii) might prove more sensitive to changes in intensity of belief, since it represents a five-point scaling of the belief from a mild or neutral belief to complete conviction, while form (i) only represents a three-point scaling of this. However, for delusions, some might argue that the belief that x is *false* (where x represents the delusional belief) is normal, and that recovery is represented by this assertion. Therefore both forms of the PQ were tested with the first subject.

Once the wording of the statement and the scaling were agreed by the patient and the interviewer, each statement was written on a 3×5 inch index card. Two further cards were added, one with MORE and the other with LESS printed on them. The procedure for the second stage, the stage of administration and scoring, was that the patient, on taking a statement card (in random order) decided whether at that moment he felt MORE or LESS certain of the belief than was stated on the card.

This procedure was followed with both subjects for their respective sets of statements at weekly intervals for ten weeks. In order to investigate the sensitivity of the measure to change, the subjects were also asked to scale other statements of the kind that would not be expected to fluctuate from week to week, for example the belief that 'the sun will rise tomorrow', 'God exists', and 'I exist'. If the scaling of these beliefs were stable, it would support the hypothesis that other changes in belief scaling (of the delusional beliefs) represented an actual change in belief intensity rather than random fluctuation in the use of the PQ alone. In order to achieve comparability of belief intensity for the control statements, normal beliefs were chosen about which subjects were certain or almost certain. Less strongly held normal beliefs may be less stable over time. For the first subject, the statement concerning the belief that the sun will rise tomorrow was expressed both in form (i) and form (ii).

One possible problem with this method of requiring a forced choice between MORE or LESS, is that a subject may think that the statement represents *exactly* his or her symptom intensity, neither more nor less. In the case of delusions this appears likely when the subject expresses absolute certainty. Phillips (1977) discusses this situation and notes that it will in general give rise to, at worst, slightly incorrect but still consistent response patterns. In this trial, PJ, while expressing informally absolute conviction, would decide on some occasions that he felt MORE certain than that x is 'definitely true' or that 'I know . . .' and on others LESS certain; in the former cases he would describe himself as 'pluperfectly convinced'. This forced choice did appear to have the effect of making the subjects discriminate carefully at the top end of the scale.

It should be noted, in relation to the technique's validity, that there are two things which the PQ might be thought of as attempting to scale: the subject's statements or the beliefs underlying the statements (Phillips 1977). Phillips argues that it is preferable to think of the PQ technique as attempting to scale the subject's actual statements of belief in a way in which the relative imprecision of everyday language does not permit, rather than assuming that it accurately reflects a state of mind.

Scoring

The subjects' responses were entered in successive columns of a table such as Tables 4.1, 4.2, and 4.3. Each block of rows represents a different set of belief statements and each row of a block a different statement of that set. (The rows of a block are arranged in decreasing

Table 4.1 *PJ's responses to six Personal Questionnaire items, form (i)*

	Week									
	1	2	3	4	5	6	7	8	9	10
(a) Dogs avoid me										
Definitely true	1	0	0	0	0	0	0	0	0	0
Probably true	1	1	1	1	1	1	1	1	1	1
May be true or false	1	1	1	1	1	1	1	1	1	1
Probably false	1	1	1	1	1	1	1	1	1	1
Definitely false	1	1	1	1	1	1	1	1	1	1
(b) People say things about me										
Definitely true	0	0	1	1	0	1	1	1	0	0
Probably true	1	1	1	1	1	1	1	1	1	1
May be true or false	1	1	1	1	1	1	1	1	1	1
Probably false	1	1	1	1	1	1	1	1	1	1
Definitely false	1	1	1	1	1	1	1	1	1	1
(c) Birds blame me and watch me										
Definitely true	1	0	1	0	0	0	0	0	0	0
Probably true	1	1	1	1	1	1	1	1	1	0
May be true or false	1	1	1	1	1	1	1	1	1	1
Probably false	1	1	1	1	1	1	1	1	1	1
Definitely false	1	1	1	1	1	1	1	1	1	1
(d) The sun will rise tomorrow										
Definitely true	0	0	0	0	0	0	0	0	0	0
Probably true	1	1	1	1	1	1	1	1	1	1
May be true or false	1	1	1	1	1	1	1	1	1	1
Probably false	1	1	1	1	1	1	1	1	1	1
Definitely false	1	1	1	1	1	1	1	1	1	1
(e) I exist										
Definitely true	1	1	1	1	1	1	1	1	1	1
Probably true	1	1	1	1	1	1	1	1	1	1
May be true or false	1	1	1	1	1	1	1	1	1	1
Probably false	1	1	1	1	1	1	1	1	1	1
Definitely false	1	1	1	1	1	1	1	1	1	1
(f) God exists										
Definitely true	0	0	0	0	0	0	0	0	0	0
Probably true	1	1	1	1	1	1	1	1	1	1
May be true or false	1	1	1	1	1	1	1	1	1	1
Probably false	1	1	1	1	1	1	1	1	1	1
Definitely false	1	1	1	1	1	1	1	1	1	1

Key: 1 = more certain; 0 = less certain.

Table 4.2 *PJ's responses to two Personal Questionnaire items, form (ii)*

	Week									
	1	2	3	4	5	6	7	8	9	10
(a) Dogs avoid me										
Know	1	0	0	0	0	0	0	0	0	0
Believe it very strongly	1	1	1	0	1	1	1	1	0	1
Believe	1	1	1	1	1	1	1	1	1	1
Have a few doubts	1	1	1	1	1	1	1	1	1	1
Doubt	1	1	1	1	1	1	1	1	1	1
(b) The sun will rise tomorrow										
Know	0	0	0	0	0	0	0	0	0	0
Believe it very strongly	1	1	1	1	1	1	1	1	1	1
Believe	1	1	1	1	1	1	1	1	1	1
Have a few doubts	1	1	1	1	1	1	1	1	1	1
Doubt	1	1	1	1	1	1	1	1	1	1

Key: 1 = more certain; 0 = less certain.

order of conviction with which the belief is held.) When a subject said that he felt MORE certain than was indicated on the card, a 1 was entered in the appropriate column, otherwise a 0 was entered. Inconsistent response patterns can be detected immediately, and the cards may either be re-presented until a consistent response is given, or scored by taking the nearest consistent pattern of responses. In this study, both subjects invariably gave consistent responses.

RESULTS

Both subjects were co-operative throughout the trial, and appeared interested in discussing their beliefs, and in making a detailed analysis of their level of conviction.

PJ's responses (forms (i) and (ii)) over ten successive weekly administrations of the PQ are given in Tables 4.1 and 4.2 respectively. While the control beliefs, 'the sun will rise tomorrow', 'I exist', and 'God exists', all remained entirely constant over the period of study, the paranoid statements were subject to some weekly fluctuation. Responses for the statement 'dogs avoid me' as measured by the two different forms of the questionnaire, are consistent between forms

Table 4.3 *RF's responses to six Personal Questionnaire items, form (i)*

	Week									
	1	2	3	4	5	6	7	8	9	10
(a) I am the Queen's son										
Definitely true	1	1	1	1	1	0	0	0	0	0
Probably true	1	1	1	1	1	0	0	0	0	0
May be true or false	1	1	1	1	1	0	0	0	0	0
Probably false	1	1	1	1	1	0	0	0	0	0
Definitely false	1	1	1	1	1	1	0	0	0	0
(b) Prince Andrew is a figment of the imagination										
Definitely true	1	1	1	1	1	0	0	0	0	0
Probably true	1	1	1	1	1	0	0	0	0	0
May be true or false	1	1	1	1	1	0	0	0	0	0
Probably false	1	1	1	1	1	0	0	0	0	0
Definitely false	1	1	1	1	1	0	0	0	0	0
(c) I did not have a car accident										
Definitely true	1	1	0	0	0	0	0	0	0	0
Probably true	1	1	1	0	1	0	0	0	0	0
May be true or false	1	1	1	0	1	0	0	0	0	0
Probably false	1	1	1	1	1	0	0	0	0	0
Definitely false	1	1	1	1	1	1	1	1	1	1
(d) The sun will rise tomorrow										
Definitely true	0	0	0	0	0	0	0	0	0	0
Probably true	1	1	1	1	1	1	1	1	1	1
May be true or false	1	1	1	1	1	1	1	1	1	1
Probably false	1	1	1	1	1	1	1	1	1	1
Definitely false	1	1	1	1	1	1	1	1	1	1
(e) I exist										
Definitely true	1	1	1	1	1	1	1	1	1	1
Probably true	1	1	1	1	1	1	1	1	1	1
May be true or false	1	1	1	1	1	1	1	1	1	1
Probably false	1	1	1	1	1	1	1	1	1	1
Definitely false	1	1	1	1	1	1	1	1	1	1
(f) God exists										
Definitely true	1	1	1	1	1	1	1	1	1	1
Probably true	1	1	1	1	1	1	1	1	1	1
May be true or false	1	1	1	1	1	1	1	1	1	1
Probably false	1	1	1	1	1	1	1	1	1	1
Definitely false	1	1	1	1	1	1	1	1	1	1

Key: 1 = more certain; 0 = less certain.

(see Table 4.1(a) and Table 4.2(b)) although form (ii) appears, as predicted, to detect more subtle changes in intensity. This does not apply to the control statement, ('the sun will rise tomorrow') (Table 4.1(d) and Table 4.2(b)) which remains constant in both forms.

The responses of the second subject (RF) are shown in Table 4.3. This man demonstrated far greater changes over the period of study, from complete conviction to complete rejection of two out of three 'delusional' statements measured. The third 'delusional' statement, 'I did not have a car accident' (Table 4.3(c)), interestingly showed greater variation in responses and by the end of the trial was not completely rejected, although it appeared to have been held *less* strongly in the early stages. As for the first subject, the control beliefs showed no change in level of conviction throughout.

DISCUSSION

It proved possible to engage two currently deluded subjects in repeated discussions of their beliefs, and to gain their co-operation in the process of constructing and administering a PQ. The subjects always gave consistent response patterns, demonstrating good internal reliability of the scale. the PQ is also shown to be sensitive to change. PJ, thought by clinicians to be severely deluded, showed some small fluctuations in his levels of conviction, although over the ten-week period, the beliefs can be said to be 'fixed', in the sense that they continued to be held at, in all cases, a level of certainty above 'may be true or false' (or, for form (ii) above the level of 'believe that'). The control beliefs, by contrast, showed absolutely no fluctuation. It is not within the scope of this trial to consider the question of why PJ's delusional beliefs fluctuated, although the changes did not appear to be closely temporally related to one potentially causative factor, the administration of injectable phenothiazines.

Sensitivity to change is demonstrated more clearly in the second subject, RF. His PQ responses ranged over the full scale, with changes that did appear to be causally related to the administration of phenothiazine medication. Indeed, in this case the repeated assessments of belief conviction took on a clinical role. It became clear after week 5 that, despite over four weeks of medication, and anecdotal reports from nursing and medical staff of wavering conviction, no consistent reduction in conviction had occurred. An increase of medication was therefore recommended, and the following week dramatic changes were evident.

However, even in this more clear-cut case where the clinical picture is of recovery, the view of delusions as discrete entities which are present or absent is challenged by these data. Thus, while the essential rejection of RF's belief 3(a) occurred in week 6, the process was not fully completed until week 7, while belief 3(c) fluctuated in intensity over some weeks, and remained as a small lingering doubt at the end. It also appears likely that cruder measures would not have detected the quite subtle differences in rate of change in RF's three delusional beliefs. Beliefs (a) and (b) are clearly related to each other, and changed at the same time, although not apparently to exactly the same extent. Belief (c) expresses a different concern, and appears to be subject to somewhat different influences. What these influences might be, whether the effects of medication, noticing contradictory evidence, or active reality testing, were beyond the scope of this trial.

Following this exploratory study, the use of the PQ with deluded subjects has been repeated and extended. Brett-Jones *et al.* (1987) reported on the use of the PQ to assess both conviction and preoccupation in nine single-case studies, in which deluded subjects were interviewed on average twelve times over approximately six months. The method of construction and administration were the same as described above. For preoccupation, which was assessed for the previous week, suggested wordings for levels of symptom intensity were offered and usually accepted. These were:

I think about these things	absolutely all of the time
"	most of the time
"	some of the time
"	occasionally
"	not at all.

Brett-Jones *et al.* (1987) found that conviction, preoccupation, and 'interference' (actions attributed to the delusions) typically did not covary. For the whole group, correlations between conviction and preoccupation and conviction and interference were very small and insignificant. The correlation between preoccupation and interference was higher ($r=0.37$, $p<0.01$). The graph (Fig. 4.1), which shows the changes in the different variables in two subjects, suggests that the variables change at different rates, reductions in conviction tending to precede reductions in preoccupation.

Chadwick and Lowe (1990) have also employed the PQ technique to assess change in delusions. They measured belief conviction and belief preoccupation in six men with persistent delusions using the method described in Brett-Jones *et al.* (1987). In addition, they employed the technique to measure the degree of anxiety experienced by

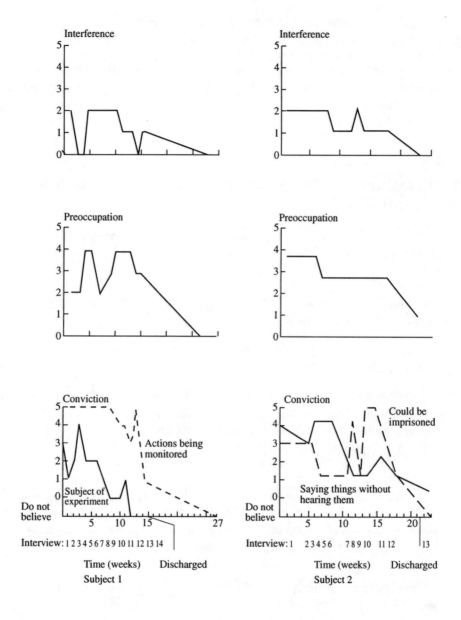

Fig. 4.1 PQ scores for preoccupation and conviction and ratings of interference in two deluded subjects over time.

the subject whilst thinking about the belief. This study was an intervention study and the results show changes in the measures, both variability in the baseline period in preoccupation and anxiety scores, although little change in conviction, and changes in all three (for some subjects) after intervention. The changes showed different patterns across subjects, and desynchrony between measures again lent support to the multidimensional view of delusions.

MEASURES TO ASSESS RESPONSIVITY OF DELUSIONS TO EVIDENCE

In viewing delusions as on continua with normal beliefs and thus potentially variably responsive to disconfirmation, two further measures were devised (Brett-Jones *et al.* 1987). Reaction to Hypothetical Contradiction (RTHC) provides a method for categorizing a subject's potential for accommodating evidence contrary to a (delusional) belief. Subjects are presented with a hypothetical but concrete and plausible piece of evidence contradictory to the belief and asked how this would affect the belief. Replies are assigned to one of four categories:

(1) evidence ignored, dismissed, or persistently denied as possible;

(2) evidence accommodated into the belief by some alteration such that the belief and evidence are now consistent;

(3) belief changes in conviction but not content;

(4) belief dropped in the face of contradictory evidence.

Accommodation, in contrast, assesses the awareness of the subject of actual occurrences contradictory to the belief, and the effect of these on the belief. Subjects are asked if anything has happened to alter their belief in any way over the past week and replies are assigned to one of five categories:

(1) no instance given, or something mentioned but with no effect on belief;

(2) some alteration in content but not in conviction or preoccupation *or* belief directly replaced by new belief;

(3) a change in conviction;

(4) a change in preoccupation;

(5) belief dropped with no replacement and subject attributes this to event.

Inter-rater reliabilities for both these measures are good.

The usefulness of these measures lies in their predictive and monitoring value. Two studies (albeit with very small numbers) have found RTHC to identify subjects most likely to change their delusions, whether following pharmacotherapy (Brett-Jones *et al.* 1987) or cognitive behavioural therapy (Chadwick and Lowe 1990). This measure has been incorporated into the MADS (Buchanan *et al.* 1993) in the belief maintenance section. Chadwick and Lowe also found that while no subject reported a single instance of accommodation during their baseline period, after the introduction of therapy subjects reported instances of disconfirmation, suggesting that the measure is useful for monitoring the effects of an intervention.

CONCLUSIONS

The assessments described in this chapter are intended primarily as clinical tools or to assist in the evaluation of therapy. The underlying model of delusions employed here is that they are in many respects like normal beliefs, in that they are multidimensional and potentially responsive to evidence and experience. Use of the measures has demonstrated that even 'fixed' delusions fluctuate to some extent, and that change along the various assessed dimensions is desynchronous. In the light of these findings, we explore more fully in the next chapter the multidimensional nature of delusions.

5 Characteristics of delusional experience*

INTRODUCTION

In Chapter 1, descriptions and definitions of delusions were reviewed. We noted then that delusions may be better viewed as phenomena which vary along a number of dimensions rather than as unidimensional phenomena. The assessments described in Chapter 4 were constructed within this framework. However, there have been remarkably few investigations of a group of deluded subjects employing such a framework. In this chapter we describe our findings from one such study.

Kendler *et al.* (1983) did follow the approach advocated here. They measured five 'dimensions' of delusional experience and posed three questions: could the dimensions be measured reliably, would they correlate highly with one another, and could factor analysis extract from these five dimensions a small number of factors that could provide an empirical basis for understanding the structure of delusional experience? The dimensions were conviction, extension (the degree to which the delusional belief involves various areas of the patient's life), bizarreness, disorganization (the extent of internal consistency, logic, and systematization), and, finally, pressure (preoccupation and concern). Rating scales were constructed to assess these dimensions, for use by an interviewer and an observer during a 45-minute semistructured psychiatric interview. Significant, but by no means high, inter-rater reliabilities were achieved (weighted kappas of 0.30 to 0.80, bizarreness proving particularly low at 0.30). The dimensions were found to be relatively independent of each other, supporting the multidimensional approach, and two factors were extracted, 'involvement' (conviction and pressure) and 'organization'.

*The content of this chapter is a revised version of two previously published papers, Garety P.A. and Hemsley, D.R. (1987). Characteristics of delusional experience. *Eur. Arch. Psychiatr. Neurol. Sci.*, **236**, 294–8, and Garety, P.A., Everitt, B.S., and Hemsley, D.R. (1988). The characteristics of delusions: a cluster analysis of deluded subjects. *Eur. Arch. Psychiatr. Neurol. Sci.*, **237**, 112–14.

However, there are problems with Kendler *et al.*'s choice of 'dimensions'. 'Extension' requires an assessment of various areas of the patient's life unlikely to be satisfactorily achieved in an interview, disorganization requires a judgement about consistency and logic, and pressure combines preoccupation and 'concern' (apparently identified evidence of the subject talking to people about the belief). It is also arguable that self- rather than observer-rating will provide more accurate information about some of these essentially private phenomena. The relatively low inter-rater reliabilities are perhaps not surprising. Some potentially important dimensions were also not assessed, such as distress and resistance.

More recently, Harrow *et al.* have described a study in which three 'major dimensions of delusional ideation' (Harrow *et al.* 1988, p. 1986) were studied in 34 psychotic in-patients. Their dimensions were: conviction, perspective (awareness of how others view the belief), and commitment ('the immediacy, importance, and urgency the patient attaches to the belief'). Commitment is assessed by combining measures of preoccupation and behaviour change. Harrow *et al.* found that while conviction correlated significantly with perspective ($r = 0.58$) and commitment ($r = 0.51$) the latter two variables were not significantly correlated ($r = 0.21$). They argue that delusions should be studied in terms of a number of dimensions, noting that on a second interview subjects often showed improvement on one dimension without a corresponding improvement on another.

Both Harrow *et al.* (1988) and Kendler *et al.* (1983) selected patients from a variety of diagnostic groups. While various claims have been made about the diagnostic significance, for the 'functional' psychoses, of different types of delusions (Cutting 1985), there is little evidence to support this, especially with respect to the formal characteristics rather than the content of the belief. Harrow *et al.* (1988) report no differences between diagnostic groups (schizophrenic, schizoaffective, and others) in their sample on the three dimensions. Cutting (1987) does present evidence for a different 'pattern' to delusions in patients with acute organic psychosis when compared with those of subjects diagnosed as schizophrenic. Thus, while it is possible that the structure of beliefs varies across diagnostic groups, this remains an empirical question. For this study, therefore, a diagnostically heterogeneous sample of deluded patients was selected, excluding those with known organic disorders.

In addition to the obvious value of gathering information on the characteristics of delusions, and considering their congruence with the formal criteria, such information may assist with a problem also outlined in Chapter 1, that of distinguishing between obsessions and delusions. One criterion thought to be important is resistance (Mayer-Gross *et al*. 1969; Mullen 1979; Oltmanns 1988) although the finding of lack of resistance in a proportion of obsessionals (Stern and Cobb 1978) was considered to weaken the usefulness of this as a distinguishing feature. Stern and Cobb, in noting a 'surprising' lack of resistance in some obsessionals, found a recognition of the senselessness of a ritual to be more characteristic. Therefore, some evidence concerning resistance and perceived senselessness in delusional subjects would clearly be valuable.

The purpose of the present study was, therefore, to describe the (subjectively assessed) characteristics of delusions in a diagnostically mixed sample, applying empirically a model of delusions as multi-dimensional.

METHOD

Subjects

The subjects were 55 psychiatric patients of the Bethlem Royal and Maudsley Hospitals described as 'deluded', regardless of diagnosis, by the psychiatrists responsible for their care. A more precise specification of the meaning of 'deluded' was deliberately omitted, in order to investigate the characteristics of the phenomenon as clinically identified, and to compare these with standard criteria. Other criteria were that the subject was aged between 18 and 65 years and not known to be suffering from an organic condition. An additional four patients were referred for inclusion: three refused to be interviewed and one was unable to complete the interview because of difficulties in concentrating on the questions.

Of the 55 subjects seen nine were out- or day-patients and 46 were in-patients. Twenty-eight (50.9 per cent) subjects were women, and the mean age of the sample was 40.3 years (SD 15.9). Thirty-five subjects were diagnosed as suffering from schizophrenia; this represents 63.6 per cent of the sample. Three subjects each (5.5 per cent) were diagnosed as suffering from schizo-affective psychosis, depression, manic depression, and hypomania. Finally, eight subjects (14.5 per cent) were either of uncertain diagnosis or thought to have a monosymptomatic delusional psychosis. Of the 46 in-patients, 31 subjects (67.4 per cent) were seen within the first month of their current admission, and 90 per cent had been in-patients for less than six months. However, three patients had been in hospital for more than 18 months. The mean length of the current admission was four months (SD 9.7). In terms of contact with psychiatric services, for the total sample, the range stretched from less than one year for eight subjects to 45 years for one individual, with the mean at 13 years (SD 11.2 years).

Measures

Characteristics of Delusions Rating Scale

A total of 11 belief characteristics drawn from the literature on delusions and obsessions were chosen for the scale. They were all characteristics capable of being assessed by an individual holding a belief, rather than by an observer; thus features such as systematization and bizarreness were not included. A visual analogue scale was devised with each characteristic represented on paper as a line which had at either end a brief description of the opposite extremes of the dimension. For the characteristic, conviction, at the end-points of the line, were the words 'believe absolutely' and 'believe not at all', while for preoccupation, the extremes of the dimension were 'thinking about it all of the time' and 'not thinking about it any of the time, ever'. The scale is presented in Table 5.1.

The subject was required to make a mark with a pen at any point on the line, to represent the extent to which that characteristic was perceived to be true of his/her belief. A visual analogue scale was chosen for this purpose since it incorporates a dimensional method of assessment, facilitates self-rating, and is easily comprehended (Clark 1984). Such scales have been used with psychotic subjects. For example, Folstein and Luria (1973) have demonstrated that a visual analogue scale provides a valid and reliable method of measuring mood states in schizophrenic subjects.

The 11 characteristics were conviction, preoccupation, interference (in terms of identifiable influence on behaviour), resistance (not liking to think about the belief), dismissibility, perceived absurdity, the extent to which the belief is thought to be self-evident, reassurance-seeking, the extent to which the belief causes worry and, separately, unhappiness, and, finally, the pervasiveness of the belief, in terms of the subject's ability to attend to other thoughts simultaneously.

The direction of the items on the scale was varied to control for response acquiescence. Indeed, in the course of the interviews the interviewer was able to detect and correct four or five subjects who appeared to be assuming that the same direction applied to all items, and were thus not attending fully to the task. Once this was pointed out, they apparently had no difficulty adjusting to the variable

Table 5.1 *Characteristics of Delusions Rating Scale*

Name: ....

Date: ....

Belief

....

1. Intensity	Believe absolutely	Believe not at all
2. Preoccupation	Not thinking about it at any time, ever	Thinking about it all of the time
3. Interference	Makes an enormous difference to what I do	Makes no difference to what I do
4. Resistance	Very much like thinking about it	Do not like thinking about it at all
5. Dismissibility	Can't dismiss it at all from my mind	Can dismiss it very easily indeed
6. Absurdity	Seems entirely sensible	Seems entirely senseless
7. Self-evident	Seems completely obvious	Seems utterly strange, implausible
8. Reassurance	Seek reassurance about it all of the time	Do not seek reassurance about it at all
9. Distress:worry	Thinking about it does not make me worry at all	Thinking about it makes me very worried
10. Distress:mood	Thinking about it makes me very unhappy	Thinking about it does not make me at all unhappy
11. Pervasiveness	Cannot think about other things at all when thinking about it	Easy to think about it and other things at the same time

direction of rating. No subdivisions were made on the line itself, but scoring was done, using a template, on a scale of $1-10$. For all items a score of 10 represented the highest degree of the assessed characteristic.

Wakefield Depression Inventory (Snaith et al. *1971)*

In addition to a self-rating of the distress (unhappiness and worry) experienced by the subject as directly related to the delusional belief, a more general assessment of depressed mood and symptomatology was made. The Wakefield Depression Inventory has been shown to be reliable, valid (that is it discriminates well between depressed and normal populations, and correlates well with another measure of depression) and brief (Snaith *et al.* 1971).

Demographic and present mental state data

These were collected from the responsible psychiatrist who responded to a short series of written questions and from the case notes. Although subjects were not fully assessed on the Present State Examination (Wing *et al.* 1974) the psychiatrists were asked to employ Present State Examination criteria to distinguish between 'partial' and 'full' delusions.

Procedure

The principal data gathering took place within the context of an interview lasting 30 minutes to one hour. After the subject had consented to the inverview he/she was asked whether anything was 'on his/her mind' or whether 'anything unusual had happened recently to him/her'. When necessary more specific probes were made with the help of information from the doctor, ward staff, or case notes. Every subject interviewed was willing to talk about his/her delusions, given appropriate reassurances about confidentiality. Once the delusion was stated, the exact wording was discussed until the subject was satisfied with it. This statement was then written clearly at the top of the rating scale.

The subject was then given the rating scale and a pen, and with the interviewer sitting beside the subject each item was explained, clarifications were given, and the subject was invited to make a mark at a point on the line to indicate the degree to which the characteristic specified represented his/her experience. Every effort was made to ensure that the subject was attending to and understood the items and thus responded accurately. Subjects were encouraged to take their time over responses and were given the opportunity to describe to the interviewer their experiences and feelings. After completing the rating scale, subjects completed the Wakefield Depression Inventory.

RESULTS

Present mental state and demographic data

The psychiatrists rated 68 per cent of subjects as fully deluded at the time they were seen, while the other 32 per cent were thought to be 'partially deluded' (using the Wing *et al.* 1974 definition). A total of 49 per cent were thought to experience auditory hallucinations and 18.5 per cent were regarded as clinically depressed. Three subjects, 5.6 per cent, were rated as currently experiencing obsessions. Some 84 per cent were being prescribed psychotropic medication, although only 37 per cent were thought to have shown a positive response to medication in the current episode; 62 per cent were said to have stable delusions, 23 per cent slowly changing, and 14.5 per cent fluctuating beliefs. With respect to marital status 65.5 per cent were single, 21.8 per cent married, 10.9 per cent divorced or separated, and 1.8 per cent widowed. Thirty-one per cent of the sample were employed, 62 per cent unemployed, and 7 per cent retired.

Wakefield Depression Inventory

Sixty per cent of the subjects achieved scores at or above the cut-off of 14 for depression on this scale. The score represents a significant degree of self-rated depressive symptoms, rather than a positive diagnosis of clinical depression (Snaith *et al.* 1971).

Characteristics of delusions

The means and standard deviations for each characteristic are given in Table 5.2. (columns 1 and 2). However, since for some items some subjects scored at one end and others at the other end (that is the scores were not normally distributed), in columns 3 to 5 the precentage of subjects scoring high (8−10), moderate (4−7), and low (1−3) is given for each item. The correlations between the characteristics were calculated using both the Spearman method and the Pearson Product Moment method. The results were similar, and the correlation matrix from the latter is given in Table 5.3.

Table 5.2 *Characteristics of delusions*

Characteristic	Total group mean score N = 55	Total group SD	Subjects with high scores (8–10) (%)	Subjects with moderate scores (4–7) (%)	Subjects with low scores (1–3) (%)
Conviction	9.1	1.8	80	20	0
Preoccupation	6.2	3.3	40	31	29
Interference	6.3	3.6	47	20	33
Resistance	7.8	3.1	69	15	16
Dismissibility	5.2	3.8	39	18	43
Absurdity	3.8	3.7	25	11	64
Self-evidentness	8.2	2.9	74	15	11
Reassurance seeking	3.6	3.1	21	21	58
Worry	6.8	3.7	56	19	25
Unhappiness	6.1	4.0	49	15	36
Pervasiveness	5.2	3.7	41	15	44

Principal components analysis

In order to investigate the intercorrelations between the various characteristics, and to estimate the extent to which some variables occur in association with each other, forming relatively independent groups of variables, a principal components analysis (PCA) was carried out.

The PCA (BMDP 1988)* was conducted on all 11 variables, employing an orthogonal (varimax) rotation of components. Four components emerged, with initial eigenvalues greater than 1 (accounting for 64 per cent of the total variance), and are shown in Table 5.4 with loadings above 0.4 given. Descriptive labels have been applied to each component.

Since independence of the components is not assumed, an oblique rotation was also conducted. This, however, yielded the same four components with very similar loadings. The correlations between the

---

*These data were initially analysed using the SPSS method, PA2, which combines an initial principal components analysis method with a subsequent factor analysis, in which an assumption about the structure of the data is made. It was this method which was reported in the Garety and Hemsley (1987) paper. In order to compare this method with a pure principal components analysis the data were re-analysed. In general, the results are very similar, yielding the same four components, although the SPSS PA2 method resulted in slightly lower loadings. The order of magnitude of variable loadings is also very similar.

Table 5.3 *Pearson product moment correlations between characteristics*

	Convic-tion	Preoccupation	Interference	Resistance	Dismissibility	Absurdity	Self-evidentness	Reassurance	Worry	Unhappiness	Per-vasiveness
Conviction	1.00										
Preoccupation	0.06	1.00									
Interference	0.11	0.28*	1.00								
Resistance	-0.04	-0.03	0.05	1.00							
Dismissibility	-0.13	-0.36**	-0.06	-0.12	1.00						
Absurdity	-0.33*	0.00	-0.01	0.28*	-0.05	1.00					
Self-evidentness	0.32*	0.27*	0.11	-0.13	-0.11	-0.49***	1.00				
Reassurance	-0.10	0.09	-0.05	-0.07	-0.11	0.20	-0.04	1.00			
Worry	0.10	0.11	0.12	0.38***	-0.11	0.21	-0.06	0.26	1.00		
Unhappiness	0.10	0.31*	0.16	0.46***	-0.36**	0.23	-0.14	0.27*	0.70***	1.00	
Pervasiveness	0.26	-0.09	-0.16	-0.18	0.32*	-0.22	0.22	-0.04	-0.26	-0.24	1.00

***$p < 0.001$; **$p < 0.01$; *$p < 0.05$.

Table 5.4 *Principal components analysis (BMDP 1988) orthogonal rotation*

	Variable	Loading	Total variance (%)
Component 1 'distress'	Resistance	0.73	
	Worry	0.83	19.5
	Unhappiness	0.82	
Component 2 'belief strength'	Conviction	0.75	
	Absurdity	−0.70	17.8
	Self-evidentness	0.72	
	Pervasiveness	0.55	
Component 3 'obtrusiveness'	Preoccupation	0.77	
	Dismissibility	−0.69	16.2
	Interference	0.51	
	Pervasiveness	−0.49	
Component 4 'concern'	Reassurance seeking	0.87	10.6

components were very low, confirming that there was little difference between orthogonal and oblique rotation.

DISCUSSION

Characteristics of delusional experience

This study found the most characteristic feature of 'delusions' to be high conviction (Table 5.2). The total mean score for conviction was 9.1 (SD 1.8), representing very strong intensity of belief. Eighty per cent of the subjects expressed high scores, and not one expressed low conviction. This was the only variable of the 11 assessed which did not elicit any low scores.

However, the responses of the subjects to the other items demonstrated a considerable degree of inter-subject variability. Aspects of beliefs thought to be typical of delusions, appear, on examination, not so typical. Thus, while many subjects (between 39 and 49 per cent) did express high levels of preoccupation, interference, dismissibility, unhappiness, and pervasiveness, many others (29 to 44 per cent) expressed low levels.

Some variables did show more clustering of scores. Suprisingly, and interestingly, more than two-thirds of the sample showed high resistance. Perhaps more predictably, subjects did not in general view their beliefs as absurd, and saw them as plainly self-evident; despite this, more than half experienced their beliefs as extremely worrying.

Delusions, then, can and do take many different forms. Nearly all will be held with 'absolute' conviction, but in addition to this some will be preoccupying, others not; some will be dismissible, others not; most will be resisted, while many will be worrying and associated with unhappiness. Most will not appear absurd; on the contrary, they will seem self-evident. Relatively few will generate the seeking of reassurance from others. The two final variables, interference and pervasiveness, were the two variables which subjects reported at the time of the assessment to be most difficult to rate. Interference required an assessment not of the belief but of associated actions, while pervasiveness required the subject to make an analysis of the degree to which his/her attention was taken up by thinking about the delusion. Interestingly, these variables showed few significant correlations with the other variables, and their loadings in the principal components analysis were lower than those of the other variables. While acting on delusions is an important aspect of delusions, it seems likely that it is not well assessed by this method.

How well do these results fit with the features of delusions described by the authorities? We found absolute conviction to be a common but not invariant feature; 20 per cent of subjects expressed only moderate conviction. Delusions are perceived as highly self-evident by three-quarters of the sample. However, in contrast to commonly accepted views, lack of resistance, at least as defined here in terms of not liking to think about the belief, is not common: 69 per cent scored high on resistance. This is not suprising if the other 'distress' measures are scrutinized; more delusions than not are greatly worrying and are perceived to cause unhappiness, a feature which figures in few definitions, although Oltmanns (1988) includes subjective distress. Most delusions are also moderately to highly preoccupying, a feature that, again, is mentioned by Oltmanns.

These data are thus consistent with the dimensional view of delusions and, of available definitions, fit best with Oltmanns (see pp. 8–9). However, the status of lack of resistance needs examining.

In this respect, the study does not assist with the problem of distinguishing between obsessions and delusions, by the standard method of appealing to the criterion of resistance (Mullen 1979). As proposed in Chapter 1, a different approach may be more fruitful, such as considering the logical structure of the phenomena. A separate study of this is warranted.

Relationships between characteristics

Few strong relationships between these individual variables were found (see Table 5.3). The strongest were the negative correlation between perceived absurdity and self-evidentness ($r = -0.49$, $p < 0.001$) and the positive correlation between the worry and the unhappiness associated with the belief ($r = 0.70$, $p < 0.001$). A number of significant, but mostly low, correlations between the variables were found. However, in general it appears that these characteristics of delusions, taken singly, are relatively independent of each other. Kendler *et al.* (1983) reported low correlations between their dimensions, and Harrow *et al.* (1988) found that two of their dimensions were poorly correlated. The study by Brett-Jones *et al.* (1987), described in more detail in Chapter 4, assessed longitudinally aspects of delusional beliefs in nine subjects. Conviction, preoccupation, and interference (behaviour thought by the subject to arise from the delusional belief) were not in general highly correlated for the whole group. Stronger correlations were found in some individual cases. Claims that delusions are multidimensional appear to be substantiated.

The relative independence of most of the variables measured here also has implications for the assessment of delusions and the assessment of change. It is not sufficient to assess one or two elements only, since the key elements do not appear to be strongly related and may not change at the same time or rate. Kendler *et al.* also make this point, noting that Hole *et al.* (1979) found that individual dimensions of delusional experience often change independently of one another during the course of a psychotic episode.

However, while individual variables were not, for the most part, strongly correlated, the principal components analysis generated four components or groups of variables (see Table 5.4). The first component, which we have labelled 'distress' has high loadings on resistance, worry, and unhappiness. The second, with high loadings on conviction, self-evidentness, pervasiveness, and, negatively, on absurdity, is named 'belief strength'. The third component, labelled 'obtrusiveness', consisted mostly of high loadings on the degree of preoccupation and interference and (negatively) of dismissibility. It also loaded, paradoxically, negatively on pervasiveness. The final component loaded mostly on reassurance seeking, and so was labelled 'concern'. All the variables therefore load on components in an understandable way, except the negative loading of pervasiveness on component three, 'obtrusiveness'. It was noted above that pervasiveness and interference were thought to be less easily rated by subjects than the other variables; this paradoxical loading may therefore reflect these difficulties rather than pointing to a significant finding.

The results of this principal components analysis suggest that there may be at least four relatively independent groups of variables underlying the 11 elements of delusional experience. With respect to the issue raised above of the need to assess a variety of dimensions adequately to assess change, taking a key variable from each of these components may be most effective. Conviction is commonly regarded as important in the assessment of change in delusions, and it has frequently been assessed alone (for example Watts *et al*. 1973; Milton *et al*. 1978). Others have recognized the importance of additionally assessing preoccupation (for example Hole *et al*. 1979; Hartman and Cashman 1983). These results suggest that it is also important to consider the subjective distress, and, to a lesser extent, the element of reassurance seeking. Behaviour may also be regarded as a separate dimension; however, it is probably not well assessed, subjectively, as attempted here with the variable 'interference'.

CONCLUSIONS

The findings of this study lend empirical support to the view of delusions as dimensional rather than all-or-nothing phenomena, and as multidimensional rather than simply expressed or measured in terms of conviction. A dimension which merits more attention is subjective distress. At the least it should be included as an outcome measure when change in delusions is being assessed; it may also relate to aetiology and treatment. More generally, however, the subjects revealed that delusions do not fit all the stereotypes. People with delusions were able to reflect on their beliefs and to give apparently reasonably consistent ratings of the beliefs' features. The extent to which we found resistance and subjective distress is at odds with the caricature of the happy lunatic contemplating his kingdom. Delusional beliefs may, it seems, demonstrate some internal consistency; they may also subjectively, at least, make sense. What then causes these phenomena?

6 Theories of the formation and maintenance of delusions*

INTRODUCTION

Theories of delusion formation are numerous, although, as noted above, very few have been subjected to experimental scrutiny. In this chapter these theories will be reviewed, together with any relevant evidence. There are two published review papers (Arthur 1964; Winters and Neale 1983) which offer fairly extensive surveys of the literature up to the early 1980s; for this reason, this review will focus on the more recent literature which is not covered by these papers. It will then be argued that models of reasoning current in cognitive psychology can be employed to formulate hypotheses of delusional belief formation and maintenance. A Bayesian model of probabilistic inference will be outlined (Fischhoff and Beyth-Marom 1983) which can be employed to test a hypothesis of a bias in belief formation in deluded subjects. However, since some of the writings at the beginning of the century provide an interesting background to current theories a selection of these will be considered first.

EARLY THEORIES OF DELUSION FORMATION

Jaspers (1913) argued that primary delusions are psychologically irreducible, arising from an unknown pathological (presumably organic) change or a change in personality. Delusions which arise understandably from preceding affects, other experiences, or hallucinations are not regarded by Jaspers as true delusions, but only delusion-like ideas. For Jaspers, therefore, an investigation into the psychological structure of delusions is unwarranted.

However, other European psychiatrists were, at about the same time, formulating quite different hypotheses. Sérieux and Capgras

---

*Part of this chapter is a revised version of Hemsley, D.R. and Garety, P.A. (1986). The formation and maintenance of delusions: a Bayesian analysis. *Br. J. Psychiat.*, **149**, 51−6.

(1909), for example, divide the 'chronic systematized psychoses' into two groups: the acquired psychoses which profoundly alter the mental functions of the subject and lead sooner or later to dementia, and the 'misinterpretative delusional states' which are based on faulty reasoning. The former originate from a disorder of perception, and hallucinations are common. Misinterpretative delusional states (which are definitionally similar to the modern-day diagnostic category of delusional disorder or paranoia), in contrast, have as their point of departure a real perception, which then, by virtue of its emotional associations, aided by erroneous inductions or deductions, takes on an intense personal significance for the subject. It is, therefore, a functional psychosis whose origin is to be found not in the action of a toxic agent but in a psychopathological predisposition arising out of an anomalous development of those cerebral association areas which subserve judgement, critical sense, and emotion. Sérieux and Capgras argue that the content of the delusion is not important diagnostically:

the nature of the delusion varies, even within the same type of psychosis, according to individual factors which make up a person's psychological orientation: personality, intellectual level, inclinations, habits, education, and the vicissitudes of life. All these intervene to steer the predisposed individual towards ideas of grandeur, persecution, mysticism or eroticism. (Sérieux and Capgras 1909, p. 108)

Dupré and Logre (1911), another two French psychiatrists, in a similar vein distinguish the origins of three delusional states. Firstly, in hallucinatory delusional states, whether acute or chronic, they suggest that the predominant disorder is one of perception. The subject regards as real perceptions what are in effect subjective products of the mind. In pure hallucinatory states a patient may embroider on what he or she regards as a genuine event in the outside world, but such interpretations are natural and logical. Sometimes, they write, one finds abundant and absurd interpretations which go beyond what should be natural interpretations of the hallucinations; nevertheless, even in these cases the hallucination always plays a major role.

The second group are misinterpretative delusional states. Dupré and Logre see these in the same terms as Sérieux and Capgras. The error is in the sphere of logic, not perception. 'The problem is not one of registering information, but of appreciating it, recognising its links with other phenomena, and establishing its relative importance and significance, in short, its interpretation.' (Dupré and Logre, 1911, p. 161).

The third category is 'confabulatory delusional states':

Those subjects affected by a confabulatory delusional state, on the other hand, are not at all worried by what they see in the outside world; nor do they feel the urge to embark on elaborate logical proofs of what is there . . . . The point of departure for their mistaken view of the world is not an idea about some external event . . . or false way of reasoning, or a false perception, but a fiction of endogenous origin, a subjective creation. Misinterpretation is a cognitive process, confabulation a poetic process. (Dupré and Logre 1911, p. 161)

This disorder derives, according to Dupré and Logre, from a condition called 'mythomania' caused by a disequilibrium of the imaginative faculty, and conceptualized as an inheritable personality disorder.

At about the same time Freud (1915) was developing his theory of paranoia and grandiosity. Freud postulated that delusions of both paranoia and grandiosity result from repressed homosexual impulses which are striving for expression. The basic unconscious thought is 'I, a man, love him' (or 'I, a woman, love her'). The anxiety stemming from this unacceptable thought causes it to be distorted and then projected, in a series of steps, to 'I, a man, hate him', to 'He hates me, so I am justified in hating him', to 'I hate him because he persecutes me'. Freud suggested that the paranoid's persecutor is always a person of the same sex who is an unconscious love object for the person. For delusions of grandiosity there is a contradiction of the homosexual impulse. The thought 'I, a man, love him' is altered to 'I do not love anyone' and then to 'I love only myself'.

These early writings incorporate views which can be separated into a number of types of explanation for the genesis of delusions: organic pathology (which gives rise to psychologically irreducible beliefs), abnormal perceptions which give rise to false accounts, faulty judgement (presumably caused by abnormal brain development), and abnormal personality either specifically given to 'mythomania' or in a more general sense accounting for the origin of delusions which symbolize the patient's unfulfilled wishes or desires. These themes are still apparent in the principal present-day theories, with an additional theme not mentioned, except in terms of Jasperian secondary delusions, that some arise directly from disturbed affect.

CURRENT THEORIES

Few would argue now that delusions are psychologically irreducible; rather they are almost universally agreed to be in some way secondary to a more basic abnormality, whether of affect, personality, unconscious wishes, perception, judgement, or some combination. Organic pathology is thought by some to be directly responsible for certain delusions. Some theories specifically concern delusions in people with the diagnoses of schizophrenia or paranoia, while others are not so restricted.

Disturbances of affect and personality

While many theorists have mentioned affect as relevant to the content of a delusion, or as an additional factor which influences its development, few have argued for a simple link from disturbed mood to abnormal belief (Winters and Neale 1983). Arthur (1964) cites Stocker (1940) who considers all delusions to be traceable to four affects, depressive, manic, anxious, and suspicious. In general, very little recent empirical work has considered the relationship between mood and delusions (Grossman 1989), perhaps because of the emphasis on schizophrenia in much of the research. Psychoanalytic accounts do, however, consider affect and as such offer the fullest motivational theories of delusions.

Jacques Lacan is regarded as the father of French psychoanalytic thinking, and, in a paper published in 1932, describes a case of a 'psychogenic psychosis'. He argues that a 38-year-old woman, 'Aimée', who stabbed a famous actress, saying that the actress had been instigating a 'scandal' against her, had developed a psychosis as a result of her personality, early experiences, and later relationships. The attack on the actress is construed as an attack on the woman's 'externalized ideal', since the freedom and social ease which writers, actresses, and women of the world reputedly possess were the very qualities which Aimée herself had dreamt of obtaining.

The most common applications of psychoanalytic concepts to delusion formation use the concept of projection, as in the case of Aimée described above. This view regards all or some delusions as symptoms which act as projections or externalizations of personal wishes, conflicts, or fears. In brief, a delusion is seen as a reflection of a personal inner, unconscious state (for example unfulfilled need, unresolved conflict) which is expressed outwardly and attributed to an external source (Winters and Neale 1983).

More recent psychoanalytic theories continue to maintain the view that delusions reflect the memories, affects, and phantasies of the individual before the psychosis overcame him/her (Freeman 1981, 1990; Nelki 1988), while not subscribing to the Freudian view that the paranoid patient is always a repressed homosexual.

According to the theory presented here, persecutory delusions are derived from wish phantasies and conflicts which come to a height immediately before the onset of an acute attack. These wish phantasies . . . existed because anxiety or guilt prevented a satisfactory outlet for instinctual wishes either directly or in sublimated form. (Freeman 1981, p. 531).

Neale (1988), more modestly, draws on psychoanalytic thinking to provide an account of one type of delusional idea. He argues that distinctly different mechanisms may be involved in the production of different types of delusional beliefs. In a chapter entitled 'The defensive functions of manic episodes', he considers grandiose delusions in mania, and argues, in line with psychodynamic thinking, that unstable self-esteem is 'the psychological predisposition' to bipolar disorder and to grandiose delusions. He further postulates that the predisposed person holds high standards of success, setting the stage for unfavourable comparisons between actuality and the ideal. He hypothesizes that the predisposed person characteristically uses pleasant phantasies as a means of coping with stress. Frequent use of pleasant phantasies to distract oneself from unpleasant events or cognitions may make the phantasies more accessible and heighten their reality (Johnson and Raye 1981), thus setting the stage for the later development of delusions. Neale argues that grandiose delusions occur, in response to a stress, whether an external event or negative cognitions, as a means of keeping distressing cognitions out of consciousness, and thus they serve a defensive function. Neale cites some indirect evidence to support this theory. A questionnaire study (Winters and Neale 1985) indicates that bipolar patients are 'defensive' and may give inaccurate reports of 'normal' self-esteem. However, he concedes that the theory is speculative, and suggests that more research is needed into the psychological causes of bipolar disorder. The work of Bentall and colleagues (Lyon *et al.* in preparation) develops Neale's work within a cognitive psychology framework and is considered below.

Psychoanalytic formulations, with theories of repression and projection, have the drawback of being difficult to subject to empirical test. However, being uninfluenced by Jaspers' theories they highlight a number of themes which may be important in understanding delusions: that content relates to pre-existing concerns, that delusions serve to reduce anxiety, and that the personality of the patient contributes to delusion formation. None of these ideas is unique to the psychoanalysts; however, they have pioneered the recognition of the meaningfulness of delusions in the face of prevailing notions of psychological irreducibility.

Neale (1988) draws on this work to formulate a speculative, if testable, account of grandiose delusions in mania. He makes the important point that different types of delusions may involve different mechanisms: a very probable and surprisingly little bruited idea.

Disturbances of perception

While many early writers have viewed some delusions as the patient's logical deduction from an altered body sensation or perception (for example Sérieux and Capgras 1909; Dupré and Logre 1911), most have provided only a very limited account of the abnormal perception itself.

Matussek (1952), drawing on gestalt psychology, considers this in more detail. He describes the change in the perceptual world of individuals undergoing a primary delusional experience as 'the splitting of individual perceptual components from their natural context'. Thus, while an ordinary person, at a railway station for example, would perceive the individual components of the scene, the train, the passengers, the station-master, etc., there would also exist a firm perceptual cohesion between them, formed by their co-ordination into the total perception of the railway station. That this comprehensive context is experienced as a whole can be seen by the surprise with which an incongruous element is perceived, such as a writing desk on the rails.

In schizophrenia, Matussek argues, this perceptual context can be more or less loosened, depending on the severity of the disturbance; in a severe disturbance, the writing desk on the rails could be perceived without surprise. How does this relate to delusion formation? Matussek suggests that when the perceptual context is weakened, individual objects acquire different properties from those which they have when the normal context prevails, leading directly, without a process of reasoning, to a delusional meaning.

Matussek's views, as noted in Chapter 3, are consistent, although emphasizing the perceptual, with other accounts of schizophrenia which descibe a disruption of the effects of expectancy and context (Fleminger, personal communication). These phenomena appear to be present in a sub-group of patients diagnosed as schizophrenic, and are plausibly causally related to the formation of some delusions.

Maher (1974, 1988) is one of the chief current proponents of a perceptual dysfunction theory of delusions. He proposes (Maher 1974) that a delusional individual suffers from primary perceptual anomalies, fundamentally biological in nature, that involve vivid and intense sensory input. There may be an experience of increased vividness of colours, or a difficulty in attending selectively to an auditory stimulus against background noise because of the increased prominence of the latter. Being prone to experience abnormal perceptual experiences, the individual seeks an explanation, which is then developed through normal cognitive mechanisms. The explanations, that is the delusions, are derived by cognitive activity that is essentially indistinguishable from that employed by non-patients, by scientists, and by people generally.

In support of this, Maher and Ross note that delusions occur in 'an enormous array of medical and psychological conditions' (Maher and Ross 1984, p. 398), and argue that this indicates that they serve some adaptive function, secondary to whatever primary disturbance has been created by the pathogenic agent.

Maher also argues that there is no evidence that deluded individuals suffer from an impairment of reasoning ability, 'apart from the inference made from the presence of the delusions themselves' (Maher 1988, p. 23). The review of the literature in Chapter 3 casts some doubt on this assertion.

Maher (1988) cites evidence from the study of normal subjects under anomalous environmental conditions, which suggests that irrational beliefs can be 'readily provoked'. Building on earlier reports of an association between hearing loss and paranoid delusions in the elderly (Cooper *et al.* 1974) and in late-onset schizophrenia (Kay *et al.* 1976), Zimbardo *et al.* (1981) proposed that a loss of auditory acuity (an unusual sensory experience), if unacknowledged, could be interpreted as other people whispering unfavourable things. In an experiment, subjects with hypnotically induced partial deafness scored higher than controls on the paranoia subscale of the Minnesota Multiphasic Personality Inventory. Johnson *et al.* (1977) also propose that delusions can arise from misattributions for unusual experiences.

Maher's account differs from Matussek's in attempting to encompass all delusions. Such a theory is plausible in those cases where an unusual sensory experience is readily detectable, and particularly has a known pathology. However, in those cases where a striking perceptual anomaly is not found (for example there is no strong evidence to suggest that paranoid people in general suffer from hearing deficits), the case is less convincing. Furthermore, in patients with psychiatric disorders it may be that the experience of anomalous percepts such as hallucinations is a less passive process than Maher suggests. Both some experiments cited in Chapter 3, in which there was evidence of deluded subjects accepting early perceptual hypotheses (McReynolds *et al.* 1964; Abroms *et al.* 1966), and current theories of hallucination formation (Slade and Bentall 1988), indicate that the cognitive style of subjects may influence the probability of experiencing perceptual anomalies.

Dupré and Logre (1911) noted that, when hallucinating, the patient mistakes for real perceptions the subjective products of the mind. Johnson (1988) discusses the interpretation involved in perception, both when 'perceiving' an actual object from ambiguous sensory input, and when attempting to discriminate between stimuli which are internally produced from those which derive from external sources (reality monitoring). As discussed in Chapter 3, Slade and Bentall (1988) draw on this work to argue that hallucinations result from a failure of the skill of reality discrimination, so that the error lies not in the information that is available but in the inferences the person makes on the basis of that information. To argue, therefore, that delusions arise from hallucinations may not be going far enough; in those cases where hallucinations appear to play a part, it may be that the delusions represent but the second stage in a process of biased inference.

Disorders of attention and consciousness

Some researchers in schizophrenia have regarded delusions as arising from disorders of mechanisms linked to perception, such as attention or consciousness. For example Payne (1970) formulated an attentional theory, in which he argued that some schizophrenics show an attention deficit characterized by over-inclusiveness, in which unjustified generalizations arise, gradually developing into delusions. Direct evidence for this is lacking.

Frith (1979, 1987) proposes, again specifically for patients with schizophrenia, that a disturbance of consciousness is involved. In 1979 he argued that the schizophrenic experiences the arrival into consciousness of percepts which would not normally be interpreted. This very arrival is important and triggers an attempt to explain and understand this unusual occurrence, using normal principles of reasoning. Frith's (1979) model thus relies heavily on the distinction between preconscious and conscious processing of information (Hemsley 1990). Frith suggests that delusions, as well as thought disorder and hallucinations, may be seen as a result of a defect in the mechanism that controls and limits the contents of consciousness. Delusions may be built up not only on the basis of hallucinatory experiences but also as a result of attention being captured by incidental details of the environment. Normally such an aspect of the situation would not reach awareness, but its registration leads to a search for reasons for its occurrence. This theory, which has much

in common with both Matussek's (1952) and Maher's (1988) pro-
posals, while plausible, is not currently supported by much empirical
evidence.

More recently, Frith (1987) suggests that a failure of the system
which monitors actions and their preceding intentions (whether
willed, that is internal, or stimulus driven, that is generated as a
response to external factors) is responsible for the positive symptoms.
'The patient fails to perceive his [*sic*] actions as a consequence of his
own will' (Frith 1987, p. 637). Thus the experience of thoughts being
initiated without any intention to initiate them would be described by
the patient as thought insertion. Another example Frith gives is of a
switch of attention caused by a willed intention which happens to be
in conflict with a current stimulus intention. If the subject has a deficit
of the monitor so that the willed intention is not recognized, this
switch requires an explanation, and for this example Frith supplies
two possibilities: (1) 'I am not in control of my actions. Some external
agent caused me to switch attention.' (delusion of passivity). (2)
'There must have been some critical signal on the channel to which
I switched. Some-one must have been talking about me.' (delusion of
reference). An experiment by Frith and Done (1989) provides results
consistent with Frith's hypothesis. Frith's is an elegant theory, which
seems to apply particularly to a sub-group of delusions, passivity
phenomena, in which the patient describes feeling that his/her actions
are controlled by someone else. It is less clear how applicable it is to
delusions in which the patient's actions are not involved. It should be
noted that Frith's theories propose that the central deficit in delusion
formation occurs at the *preconscious* processing stage, while other
theories (such as those which involve disorders of perception and
judgement) emphasize a conscious search for explanation.

Neuropsychological causes

Cutting (1985, 1991) asks whether the cause of delusions can be
formulated in neuropsychological terms. He proposes that delusions
in some schizophrenics are caused by either left temporal or right
parietal dysfunction. He cites evidence that there is a statistical
association between left temporal lesions and schizophrenia with
prominent paranoid delusions and delusions of reference (Toone *et al*.
1982), suggesting that in these cases delusion formation is facilitated
by affective associations being made to previously neutral stimuli.
Cutting links this theory with Bleuler's (1906) that enhanced emotional attachment to an idea predisposes to paranoid delusions.

Cutting further argues that right parietal damage encourages delusion formation through its effect on perception. He cites two types of abnormal beliefs, the Capgras phenomenon and anosognosia, as vivid illustrations of this. The Capgras phenomenon, or the illusion of doubles, is the delusional negation of the identity of a familiar person. Anosognosia is the belief that a physical disability (indisputably present in the subject) does not exist. Cutting quotes papers which link these beliefs with organic brain damage, causing visual agnosia, implicating an underlying perceptual disorder. Ellis and Young (1990) have also reported that disorders in facial recognition are found in patients suffering from delusional misidentification.

While ingenious, the work on anosognosia seems more relevant for a subset of delusions found in people with known organic damage than for schizophrenics generally. It does appear possible that right-hemisphere abnormalities are implicated in Capgras delusions. These beliefs are by no means restricted to patients with a diagnosis of schizophrenia. They have been reported as occurring in the context of a dementing illness and Fleminger (personal communication), reviewing the literature, argues that 'there can be little doubt of the association of Capgras' syndrome, as well as other delusional misidentification syndromes, with organic cerebral disorder'. However, Fleminger goes on to argue that in schizophrenia, where the extent of the organic impairment of the perceptual system is likely to be small, delusional misidentification will only arise if 'powerful top-down' effects (that is, a bias to being excessively influenced by prior expectations rather than immediate stimuli) are able to disrupt the potentially unstable perceptual system. He concludes 'in the functional psychoses, strong psychological forces will be needed to disrupt the relatively normal perceptual system'. Fleminger thus proposes that a cognitive bias influences the processing of data in a perceptual system which may already be vulnerable, but not defective.

A number of papers have recently considered frontal lobe damage in relation to delusions (Butler and Braff 1991; O'Carroll 1992). For example, Benson and Stuss (1990) describe five case studies of organic delusional syndromes featuring frontal lobe damage. Arguing from these cases that reality testing is dependent on competent frontal lobe functioning, they contend that the frequent association of schizophrenic delusions with prefrontal malfunction suggests organic involvement. In contrast, however, Liddle and Morris (1991) assessed 43 chronic schizophrenic patients on a battery of tests allegedly sensitive to frontal lobe dysfunction. No significant correlations emerged between the test results and scores on the reality distortion (delusions and hallucinations) syndrome. However, even if a location in the brain is identified which is associated with certain types of delusions, this does not obviate the need to consider which psychological processes are disrupted; indeed Shallice *et al.* (1991) have argued recently that the attempt to understand the nature of the processing impairment in schizophrenia should precede the attempt to localize it.

Abnormalities of reasoning

In Chapter 3 the experimental literature on reasoning in deluded subjects and in patients diagnosed as schizophrenic was reviewed. Some of the theories of delusion formation or maintenance which posit a reasoning bias have thus already been considered. In this section, besides briefly referring to these theories, other theories of delusion formation and maintenance which incorporate a reasoning abnormality will be described, and we will then propose a new framework within which to test hypotheses.

The early literature cited above (Sérieux and Capgras 1909; Dupré and Logre 1991) proposed that some delusions arise from errors in the sphere of logic. This view was more explicitly formulated by Von Domarus in 1944, subjected to experimental scrutiny in the 1950s and early 1960s, and then widely thought to have been refuted by a lack of supporting evidence (for example Maher 1988). Perhaps as a consequence of this few psychological theories incorporating a reasoning bias have been formulated in recent years, despite the retention of the idea of inferential failure in psychiatric definitions.

Heilbrun (1975) has developed a theory of paranoia which combines information processing with social learning approaches. He maintains that persistent experiences of aversive control by the mother facilitates the learning of either of two styles of cognitive adaptation in the child: the open style, which is characterized by social approach strategies and perceptual vigilance, and the closed style, which involves social withdrawal and perceptual defence. These styles produce different kinds of delusional thinking. Open-style thinkers process information by a broad search of stimuli, selective perception of negative cues, premature attribution of meaning, and erroneous projection of negative evaluative information to others. For closed-style thinkers, evaluative information is actively avoided to protect a fragile self-esteem. Heilbrun and associates have conducted a series of studies to assess various aspects of the model (Heilbrun 1975; Heilbrun and Bronson 1975; Heilbrun and Heilbrun 1977). These have all been conducted with normals, who are assigned to groups according to the cognitive styles of adaptation. Winters and Neale (1983) comment that while there have been findings in a number of studies that subjects with open and closed styles of adaptation are differentiated on a number of behaviours, relating these findings to delusion formation is problematic. Furthermore, the maternal child-rearing practices of mothers of schizophrenics have not been demonstrated to comply with the model. However, Heilbrun's ideas concerning different styles of information processing among different groups of deluded subjects are of interest theoretically and have interesting echoes in some more recent works such as that of Bentall and colleagues (see below).

Reed proposes that (primary) delusions arise because the schemata which are employed to organize the input and output of meanings have 'shifted their interrelations' (Reed 1988, p. 154). He argues that cognitive *processes* are unimpaired, but that cognitive *structures* have shifted. In support of this, Reed cites Bannister's (1960) work in Personal Construct Theory, in which the schizophrenic is thought to be continually denied the expectations generated by his/her constructs, which results in a loosening in the normal organization of cognitive structures, accounting for the symptom of thought disorder. This Reed likens to his notion of a shift in the relationships between schemata. Radley (1974) also discusses Bannister's theory, suggesting that paranoid thinking may arise from a predisposition to employ 'cognitively simple' constructs, which are tightly organized but idiosyncratic. Such a thinking style will respond to apparent inconsistencies, not by employing superordinate constructs which seek to resolve the inconsistency but by forming non-integrated successive, contrasting impressions or choosing a construction which applies to only one facet of the situation. 'This might reflect an attempt by the individual to establish a coherent impression . . . by focusing on one aspect . . . and "ignoring" evidence to the contrary' (Radley 1974, p. 321). The paranoid individual is seen as motivated to deal with invalidation by reallocating incompatible elements with minimum change to the overall structure in the construct system. (This idea has echoes of Quine's (1953) views; see p. 20). If, however, this strategy fails, and new evidence continually appears which cannot be integrated, the constructs themselves may have to be altered. Bannister's (1960) hypothesis is that this reorganization takes the form of progressive loosening of the associations between a person's constructs so that the predictions become less precise, and the thinking changes from the tightly organized delusional thinking of the paranoid to the loosely structured thinking characteristic of thought disorder.

These ideas are interesting in proposing a two-stage process in which delusions result from an early strategy of adaptation to a thinking style (or reasoning bias) and, when that fails, thought disorder results. Of course, for some this symptom pattern does not occur, and they remain chronically deluded; this is not explained by the model. As for so many of these (often plausible) theories, direct experimental evidence is weak.

In Chapter 3, recent work by Hemsley (1987) was described. Hemsley argued that weakening of the influence of stored memories of regularities of previous input on current perception occurs in schizophrenia. Thus schizophrenics are less able to make use of the redundancy and patterning of sensory input to reduce information processing demands. Hemsley (1990) develops his argument to speculate on the formation of delusions in schizophrenics. He notes that people have a tendency to search for causal explanations when events violate expectations. He further notes that temporal order and contiguity indicate causal relationships, taken together with covariation information (that is information about past regularities). If schizophrenia is characterized by awareness of aspects of the environment not normally attended to and a reduction of the influence of past regularities on present perception, then, he argues, abnormal causal relationships (delusional beliefs) may be inferred on the basis of a single co-occurrence.

Schneider (1930) put this clearly when he noted that 'meaningful connections are created between temporarily coincident external impressions, an external impression with the patient's present condition, or perception with thoughts which happen to be present, or events and recollections happening to occur in consciousness about the same time'. Similarly Arieti observed 'patients see nonfortuitous coincidences everywhere' (Arieti 1974, p. 231). Matussek quotes a patient as saying 'out of these perceptions come the absolute awareness that my ability to see connections had been multiplied many times over' (Matussek 1952, p. 96). For example, objects showing certain qualities which had become prominent were seen as being linked in some significant way. Such feelings of relatedness, based on temporal or spatial contiguity between experiences, may proceed to an assumption of a causal relationship between them. Meehl (1964) (quoted in Eckblad and Chapman 1983), claims that schizophrenia-prone individuals 'entertain the possibility that events which, according to the causal concepts of this culture, cannot have a causal relation with each other, might nevertheless do so'.

The 'Immediacy Hypothesis' of Salzinger (1984) bears some similarity to Hemsley's theory: it states that the behaviour of schizophrenic individuals is controlled by stimuli immediate in their environment. Salzinger further argues that responding to immediate stimuli means responding to stimuli in isolation, 'typically it is the context — that is the other stimuli present either at the same time or before — that gives accurate meaning' (Salzinger 1984, p. 249), and that this will lead to errors, such as delusions. 'A delusion is almost an operational definition of responding to stimuli out of context' (Salzinger 1984, p. 249).

Kaney and Bentall (1989) and Bentall *et al.* (1991) (discussed in Chapter 3) have found attributional style differences between deluded subjects with persecutory delusions and non-deluded subjects. Paranoid subjects show a systematic tendency to blame other people if something goes wrong, whereas they attribute good outcomes to themselves. Bentall and colleagues have suggested that paranoid subjects have an exaggerated 'self-serving bias' and have gone on to suggest that paranoid patients suffer from defended low self-esteem. Persecutory delusions, they suggest, serve the function of avoiding the presence of negative self-referent thoughts in consciousness (Lyon *et al.* in preparation). At present, however, this research is correlational and it is not clear what role attributional biases play in the formation (as opposed, perhaps, to the maintenance) of delusions.

Chapman and Chapman (1988) discuss Maher's theory of the role of anomalous experiences in the genesis of delusions, and comment that if delusions are reasonable interpretations of such experiences, subjects with similar experiences should have similar beliefs. They examined the relationship of beliefs of experience in 'psychosis-prone' students (identified by high scores on the Magical Ideation Scale (Eckblad and Chapman 1983) and the Perceptual Aberration Scale (Chapman *et al.* 1978)) and found that subjects responded to similar experiences with beliefs that ranged from the normal to the fully delusional. They found some cases in which a delusion was the 'clear result' of an anomalous perceptual experience because acceptance of the veridicality of the experience demanded, or almost demanded, a delusional belief. Other subjects reported delusions or aberrant beliefs which had no apparent relationship to any unusual experiences. Still others reported delusions that had some relation to their unusual experiences, but yet were not necessary, nor even reasonable interpretations of those experiences.

Chapman and Chapman describe a number of accounts given by subjects of 'hearing voices', and conclude that the data indicate that a voice experience is subject to radically different interpretations ranging from the normal to the slightly aberrant to the delusional. They doubt, on the basis of the descriptions given, that those who gave the delusional accounts were subject to more vivid perceptual events.

They also argue that anomalous perceptual experiences are not necessary for the formation of a delusion. Some subjects developed aberrant or delusional beliefs in response to experiences which would not be considered anomalous by most people, such as interpreting shadows at night as indicating the actions of spirits.

Chapman and Chapman go on to attempt to account for the apparently unreasonable conclusions reached by some subjects by introducing a concept labelled 'cognitive slippage', to refer to a less severe form of the formal thought disorder found in some schizophrenic patients. As some schizophrenic patients reason so badly about most problems in their lives, it would, they assert, be unexpected if they reasoned more accurately about delusional topics. The Chapmans note that their interviewers were struck by the upsurge of cognitive slippage when subjects talked about psychotic experiences, including delusions. They expressed themselves vaguely, became tangential, jumped inappropriately from one topic to another, and had difficulty finding the right choice of words. Delusional patients seemed to constrict the information used in reaching a conclusion, ignoring or giving inadequate weight to other experiences, some of which may contradict the delusional belief. A person who interprets shadows as reflecting spirit influences is failing to incorporate the fact that shadows are commonplace and result from the play of light on objects.

Chapman and Chapman note that Maher regards the failure of subjects to ignore conflicting information as similar to the processes involved when scientists stick tenaciously to favoured hypotheses. They argue that although scientists, like delusional patients, ignore contradictory evidence in reaching their conclusions, delusional patients clearly ignore more obvious and relevant information than scientists. Delusional patients deny well established facts of physical reality that they and others have experienced all their lives. Thus, delusional patients do not show a qualitatively unique kind of error but instead accentuate a normal error tendency to a point of gross deviancy. They argue that the reasoning bias of delusional patients lies in selecting and focusing more often on stimuli that are strong or prominent by normal standards, neglecting weaker stimuli. This view is similar to Salzinger's immediacy hypothesis and compatible with Hemsley's views about the tendency of schizophrenics to fail to take account of past learned regularities.

While challenging Maher's theory, the Chapmans do not reject it entirely. They suggest that his account of delusional persons reasoning in a normal way has its greatest appeal for subjects who do not show formal thought disorder, such as patients with pure paranoia.

None of these theories specifically addresses the question of whether the *maintenance* of the delusional belief involves a process of abnormal reasoning. Cameron (1951) suggested that paranoid patients disregard information incongruent with their delusional systems, but few others have raised this issue.

Discussion

Delusions are clearly complex phenomena, and it is likely that a number of factors contribute to their formation and maintenance. It is also likely, as noted above, that different types of delusions involve different mechanisms. That personality, affect, self-esteem, and unconscious wishes play a part in some is highly probable; however, an additional or even primary abnormality appears to be implicated in a large number of these beliefs, perhaps especially in those where a mood disorder does not predominate. Some of this latter category may be the result of a brain insult or toxic state; other beliefs, where no organic abnormality can be detected, have as their prime candidates for causation abnormalities of perception or of judgement. However, we have seen how perception is not judgement-free, and that experiencing abnormal percepts may be accounted for, at least in part, by a judgemental bias. This fact, combined with some direct evidence for biased judgement (see Chapter 3), strengthens the argument for further investigations of reasoning in deluded subjects.

An empirical study of reasoning in deluded subjects will be described in the next chapter. Before reporting on the study, however, some theoretical issues warrant exploration. One major problem with studying reasoning, which beset the investigators of the Von Domarus principle, is setting a norm for correct reasoning. A model for this, which leads to an experimental paradigm, will be proposed in the next section.

A BAYESIAN MODEL OF THE FORMATION AND MAINTENANCE OF DELUSIONS

In Chapter 2 a model of rationality which required of people adherence to the methods of formal logic was rejected. It was clear that reasoning is not restricted to logic, and that people typically employ a number of heuristic devices which guide expectations and assist reasoning, although they may also lead to errors (Ross and Anderson 1982). Making inferences, as Alloy and Tabachnik (1984) argued, results from a combination of the strength of the prior belief and the current situational information. This also applies to changing or maintaining hypotheses.

In order to study how people reason Fischhoff and Beyth-Marom (1983) have argued that a normative model is needed to provide a conceptual framework within which the actual performance of people can be studied. They propose that Bayesian inference provides a general framework for evaluating beliefs, and it is possible to describe a person's consistency with, or departures from, the theoretical model. They identify a set of logically possible deviations from Bayesian behaviour and review the research literature to see whether these possibilities correspond to observed behaviour in the normal population. It is proposed here that this approach may also be usefully applied to the study of reasoning in deluded patients.

From the Bayesian perspective, knowledge is represented in terms of statements or hypotheses, H_i, each of which is characterized by a subjective probability, $p(H_i)$, representing one's confidence in its truth. Bayes' theorem then governs the way in which the strength of one's belief in a hypothesis should be revised in the light of new information or data (D). In its simplest form, the theorem deals with the implications of the datum (D) for the relative likelihoods of a hypothesis (H) and its complement (not-H). In such cases Bayes' theorem states that

$$\frac{p(H/D)}{p(\bar{H}/D)} = \frac{p(D/H)}{p(D/\bar{H})} \cdot \frac{p(H)}{p(\bar{H})}.$$

Reading from right to left, the three terms in the formula are: (1) the prior odds that H and not-H ($\bar{H}$) are true in the light of all that is known before the receipt of D; (2) the likelihood ratio, representing the information value of D with respect to the truth of H; and (3) the posterior odds that H is true in the light of all that is known after the receipt of D. This approach has the advantage, for studying delusions, of incorporating the level of the prior belief explicitly in the inferential process.

Fischhoff and Beyth-Marom (1983) point out that Bayesian inference is a normative scheme and that it is logically possible to deviate from optimal Bayesian performance in a number of ways. This therefore provides a scheme for categorizing different types of judgemental processes and considering whether a particular form of deviation is characteristic of a given group of people, such as deluded subjects.

Fischhoff and Beyth-Marom suggest a number of potential biases that can occur in hypothesis evaluation. These may occur at the stages of:

(1) the identification of the data sources which are most useful for discriminating between competing hypotheses;

(2) the assessment of the implications of an observed datum *vis-à-vis* the truth of competing hypotheses;

(3) the aggregation of the implications of different data with an overall appraisal of the relative likelihood of the truth of the hypothesis;

(4) the selection, based on that appraisal, of the appropriate course of action.

For a given belief, a deluded subject may therefore demonstrate deviation from the Bayesian model at one or more of the above stages. A Bayesian framework has been used for the experimental study of the inferential style of one clinical population, obsessional patients, by Volans (1976). She reported that obsessional subjects, when compared with phobic and normal groups, and after partialling out neuroticism, differed with respect to the amount of evidence they required prior to making a decision: the obsessional group required more information at this stage.

OTHER CONSIDERATIONS

Content-specificity

Some of the experimental studies described in Chapter 3 used materials apparently relevant to subjects' delusions, such as the Brennan and Hemsley (1984) study of illusory correlations, while others (for example McReynolds *et al.* 1964) employed materials without any apparent relevance. Some of the literature reviewed in this chapter has suggested that the affective tone of the content of the material may influence delusion formation (for example Cutting 1985). For this reason, it is proposed that in an experimental study of reasoning in deluded subjects it is of interest to study performance with 'neutral' material (hypothesized to be without affective loading for the subjects). If a bias, when compared with controls, is absent with this material, obviously an independent or interacting content-specific bias may still be found. However, a bias with neutral material might reflect a more generalized or fundamental judgemental abnormality.

Sub-group specificity and mood specificity

In addition to the issue of content-specificity, there is also the question of sub-group specificity in any reasoning bias. It has been argued (Chapman and Chapman 1988) that Maher's theory may apply best to subjects who do not show formal thought disorder, such as patients with pure paranoia. However, these are very often people who do not give accounts of experiencing any very obvious perceptual anomalies such as hallucinations. Neale (1988) proposed that patients with bipolar disorder may form delusions involving different mechanisms from those involved in schizophrenia. While there is considerable literature concerning cognitive processing in depression, there is little literature describing studies of reasoning in deluded subjects with a primary affective disorder. In the study reported in the next chapter, it was decided to restrict the investigation to subjects who did not have a primary affective disorder or known organic pathology, and to compare subjects with a clear diagnosis of schizophrenia with those with pure paranoia or delusional disorder.

CONCLUSIONS

On p. 82 it was concluded that delusions are complex phenomena, and that it is likely that a number of factors contribute to their formation and maintenance. For some delusional beliefs, abnormalities of perception or of judgement (which may not be independent) were thought to play a causal role, a view to which support is lent by the experimental evidence cited in Chapter 3. It is proposed here that reasoning in deluded subjects can be studied employing a Bayesian normative framework, and that a 'neutral' content task may extend our understanding of putative biases in patients with diagnoses of schizophrenia and of paranoia. Such a study is described in the next chapter.

7 Reasoning in people with delusions*

INTRODUCTION

A review of rationality and reasoning in deluded and schizophrenic subjects in Chapter 3 indicated that there was some evidence for a reasoning bias in deluded subjects. Theories of delusion formation just reviewed (Chapter 6), which are compatible with the evidence, such as Chapman and Chapman's (1988), do not, however, propose any very specific theoretical framework for evaluating reasoning in deluded subjects. In addition, given the reasoning biases found in the normal population and the growing acceptance of delusions as continuous with normal beliefs, we have argued that it may be productive to investigate this, employing a framework which has been applied to normal beliefs and for which experimental methods of investigation have been already devised. A Bayesian model of probabilistic reasoning has therefore been proposed.

A PILOT STUDY

Introduction

Huq *et al.* (1988) conducted a study, employing a Bayesian framework, which served as a pilot study for the experiment to be described later in this chapter. It was hypothesized, on the basis of the clinical phenomena and experimental findings, that intensity of conviction, fixity of belief, and rapid decision-making might be greater in deluded than control subjects. Thus, the pilot study investigated whether deluded subjects showed any biases in decision-making, using 'neutral' material, deviating not only from a Bayesian norm but

*In this chapter we present revised versions of two previously published papers: Huq, S.F., Garety, P.A., and Hemsley, D.R. (1988). Probabilistic judgments in deluded and non-deluded subjects. *Q. J. Exp. Psychol.*, **40A**, 801–12, and Garety, P.A., Hemsley, D.R., and Wessely, S. (1991). Reasoning in deluded schizophrenic and paranoid patients: biases in performance on a probabilistic inference task. *J. Nervous Mental Dis.*, **179**, 194–201.

also from a normal control group and a control group of psychiatric patients.

The basic paradigm

In a typical experiment on probability judgements (Phillips and Edwards 1966) subjects are shown containers holding a large number of poker chips of two different colours, such as red and green. Containers labelled A and B have red and green chips in a particular ratio, for example 70 green/30 red, or the reverse. Subjects are informed of the proportions, and containers are removed from view. Subjects are then told about the prior probabilities, that is that either of the containers is equally likely to be chosen. The initial prior probabilities are thus always 50A:50B. One of the containers is then chosen, and a sample is drawn from the chosen container. The experiment is continued, with samples from one being drawn sequentially and samples replaced. The subject's task is to work out whether the experimenter is drawing from container A or container B. S/he may also have the additional task of indicating at each stage in the sequence estimates of the probabilities that each container had been chosen. Under different conditions the number and sequence of draws will vary, according to predetermined criteria. There is an optimal 'rational' strategy for performance on these tasks. At each stage, Bayes' theorem can be used to compute the likelihood of a given container having been selected, given the data presented. Edwards (1982) notes that the normal population is consistently conservative in the estimates given in such a task.

Method

Materials and measures

Eight jam jars, each containing 100 coloured beads, constituted the stimulus material. There were four pairs of jars; in every pair there were, in each jar, two sets of coloured beads in equal and opposite proportions; for example in set W jar A contained pink and green beads, in the ratio 85 pink and 15 green beads and jar B contained green and pink beads, in the ratio 85 green and 15 pink beads. The other sets were identical, except that they contained beads of different colours.

In order to register probabilities of hypothesis and event predictions, subjects were provided with a response board. This is described fully in Huq *et al.* (1988).

Procedure

Before beginning each condition, subjects were asked to read the relevant written instructions. These were clarified with the subject, who then practised use of the response board. Emphasis was placed on three points: that draws would be taken from the same jar for all trials to be given with the same set; that beads would be replaced in the same jar after each draw; and that subjects were allowed as many trials as they needed to be completely sure as to which jar had been chosen.

There were four experimental conditions:

Condition 1: A YES−NO response mode was used. Subjects were shown beads drawn from one (hidden) jar, following a predetermined sequence. They were asked to indicate whether or not they required more draws before they came to a decision as to which jar had been chosen, and when they indicated they had decided were asked to say which jar they thought the draw/draws came from.

Condition 2: A YES−NO response mode was employed in the same way as for Condition 1. Beads from one jar were shown in a predetermined sequence, and subjects requested as many draws as they wished before reaching a decision. In addition, before each draw, subjects were required to indicate their estimates of the probability of a given colour bead being about to be drawn by using the response board.

Condition 3: A probabilistic response mode was used in this condition. After each draw, subjects were required to indicate the relative probabilities that they attached to the draw having come from either of the two jars, using the response board. No estimations about individual beads were required.

Condition 4: This condition required the subject to give estimations concerning the probability of a given colour bead being drawn prior to each draw, as in Condition 2, and then, following each draw, subjects were asked to indicate the relative probability of the draw having come from either of the two jars, as in Condition 3.

Subjects

The experimental subjects were 15 deluded (D) schizophrenics. The criteria for selection were:

(1) a clear diagnosis of schizophrenia, as determined by the psychiatrist responsible for the patient's care;

(2) current delusions at a high level of intensity, as assessed from ratings made by subjects for a separate study (Garety and Hemsley 1987, as reported in Chapter 5);

(3) absence of formal thought disorder (assessed by the psychiatrist).

The 10 patients forming the non-deluded psychiatric control group (ND) were of various diagnoses: depression (2), manic depression (4), phobia (2), anxiety state (1), and eating disorder (1), and were required to show no evidence of delusions. In addition, in view of Volans' (1976) results, obsessional subjects were excluded.

The normal control group consisted of 15 volunteers who were asked to confirm that they had no psychiatric history.

There were no significant differences between groups for either age or score on the Mill Hill Vocabulary Scale.

Dependent variables

1. *Draws to decision.* The average of draws taken on all four conditions to reach a decision as to which jar had been chosen, excluding the initial draw.

2. *Initial certainty level* following the first draw of Conditions 3 and 4. The subject's probability estimate was subtracted from that predicted by the Bayesian model.

3. *Event estimations.* These were calculated as deviations from the Bayesian norm in the subjects' estimates of the likelihood of a given colour bead appearing on the first draw. As subjects had no evidence on which to base their estimate, the rational (Bayesian) estimate would be 50 per cent for any set of two beads. The average of Conditions 2 and 4 was taken.

4. *Errors in decision-making.* Very few errors were made (D=6, ND=1; N=3). The findings for the other dependent variables are presented in Table 7.1.

Two-way analyses of variance were carried out to examine group differences on draws to decision and initial certainty level. In neither

Table 7.1 *Mean scores on dependent variables for the three groups*

Groups	Draws to decision		Initial certainty		Event estimation	
	Mean	SD	Mean	SD	Mean	SD
D	1.22	1.57	6.40	17.37	67.79	21.22
ND	3.58	3.51	20.58	12.38	55.36	13.12
N	2.60	1.17	19.87	9.37	59.30	13.99

case was the order effect or group by order effect significant. A significant group effect on both draws to decision $F(2,28)=3.35$, $p<0.05$, and initial certainty level, $F(2,28)=4.87$, $p<0.05$, was found. The difference between the normal and the deluded group on the former was significant ($t(28)=1.7$, $p<0.05$, one-tailed). Because of the large variance in the deluded group on the latter variable, the results were checked by means of a Fisher's Exact Test. The non-deluded and normal controls were grouped together, and the resulting two groups were divided according to whether the deviation scores were negative or positive, that is expressing under- or over-confidence. There was a highly significant association between group membership and likelihood of a negative (over-confident) deviation score ($p<0.005$). For event estimation, the tendency for the deluded group to express higher probability estimates than the other two groups was not statistically significant (Kruskal−Wallis test, $\chi^2(2)=2.56$, $p=0.28$).

Discussion

The results of this pilot study suggested that on a neutral task deluded subjects require less evidence than normals or non-deluded psychiatric patients before reaching a decision. They also express higher levels of certainty after the first item of information is presented than either of the two control groups. (Indeed, the two measures were highly correlated ($r=0.58$, $p<0.0001$).) These results are consistent with the research reviewed in Chapter 3.

However, in reaching rapid decisions it is not clear at this stage what underlies the bias. Are the deluded subjects experiencing a disruption of 'gestalt' perception so that the part is taken to equal the whole (Cutting 1985)? Or does this rapid decision-making stem from an over-emphasis on present stimuli, neglecting past learning (Hemsley 1987)?

Interpreting these results presents some other difficulties. For 'draws to decision' the deluded subjects' average decision point was after the presentation of 2.22 items of information (that is after the first draw, which all subjects received, plus the mean 1.22 draws additionally requested). Under all conditions the first two draws selected beads of the same colour, and at this point the objective probability that the jar containing predominantly beads of that colour had been chosen was 97 per cent. Thus it may be argued that the deluded sample reached a decision at an objectively 'rational' point. It may further be argued that the two control groups were over-cautious, the normal sample reaching a decision at between on average 99.5 per cent certainty on Conditions 1 and 3 and 97 per cent certainty on Conditions 2 and 4, and the psychiatric control group at between on average 99.9 and 97 per cent certainty. There was, however, considerable variability within the experimental group. Seven of the deluded sample (47 per cent) made the decision, on *all* conditions, after the very first draw, at the point of 85 per cent probability, something that occurred in only one of the 25 controls.

The related measure, 'initial certainty', yields a consistent picture. Here, again, a group effect was found, the deluded group expressing higher levels of conviction from the outset than the other two groups. In this respect, again, the deluded subjects are more 'rational' according to the Bayesian model than the other two groups — whereas all groups are over-cautious in their estimates, this is more marked in the two control groups. This 'conservatism' is consistent with the Phillips and Edwards (1966) original finding, and also with a wealth of studies reported by Edwards (1982), and is particularly marked when, as in this case, the task is easy (Lichtenstein *et al.* 1982). Again within the experimental group there were marked differences: six of the deluded groups were over- not under-confident in their certainty levels, while over-confidence did not occur in any of the 25 controls.

The deluded subjects exhibited over-confidence in 'event estimation', estimates of the likelihood of a given colour bead appearing on the first draw. The correct probability was always 50 per cent; the normal group averaged 59 per cent, the non-deluded controls 55 per cent, and the deluded group 68 per cent. Even though the difference between the groups was not statistically significant, the deluded group again expressed higher levels of conviction. In this case, the deluded group's performance appears less normative than that in the control groups, in contrast to their performance on draws to decision and initial certainty. The direction of the effect is, however, consistent with these other measures.

The results of this study did not indicate any distinct sub-groups in the deluded sample, although the variability in responses was large; however, the number of deluded subjects was relatively small and the selection of the sample did not specify sufficiently rigorously the characteristics of subjects, nor provide data on other aspects of the subjects' current symptomatic state. The results were consistent with the hypothesis that some, but not all, deluded subjects show a reasoning bias characterized by rapid and over-confident decision-making.

The experiment only tested aspects of hypothesis formation, and not belief maintenance/change. It is possible to modify the procedure to incorporate the latter. This was therefore undertaken in the main study.

REASONING IN DELUDED PATIENTS: A STUDY OF PERFORMANCE ON A PROBABILISTIC INFERENCE TASK

Introduction

The Huq *et al.* (1988) study indicated that deluded subjects, as a group, have a tendency to make rapid and over-confident decisions, but that this bias may be confined to a sub-group of deluded subjects. The literature reviewed in Chapters 3 and 6 suggests that subjects with delusions in the absence of other symptoms (that is with paranoia or delusional disorder) may be fruitfully compared with deluded subjects in whom other symptoms are present (subjects with a diagnosis of schizophrenia). It was this that was attempted. Two alternative hypotheses arise concerning this from the literature. Firstly, Chapman and Chapman (1988) argue that schizophrenics would be more likely to show reasoning abnormalities. On the other hand, where delusions are regarded as a normal attempt to account for abnormal experience (Frith 1979; Maher 1988) a reasoning bias may be more likely in patients who give no evidence of abnormal experiences, such as hallucinations (that is those with delusional disorder).

In addition to studying whether the pilot study results would be replicated with a differently constituted and larger sample of deluded subjects (and compared with a more homogeneous psychiatric control group known to be free of a history of delusions), the procedure was modified to incorporate a test of belief change. As noted above, very few theorists have considered the issue of belief change in delusions, although the definitions emphasize their incorrigibility. The second condition was therefore designed to test subjects' readiness to change a (strongly held) hypothesis when confronted with counter-evidence.

Method

Material and measures

The present study employed the same basic paradigm, equipment, and method as the pilot study. The results are compared with Bayesian norms and also with the performance of a psychiatric (anxious) and a normal control group.

Since there were only two conditions rather than four, four jam jars, each containing 100 coloured beads, constituted the stimulus material, divided into two pairs. In all other respects, they were as described above. The ratio of beads of one colour to beads of the other was the same: 85:15.

Procedure

Data lists were prepared in advance. This ensured that every subject would be shown the same sequence of colours in each condition. The sequence of draws in the two conditions (where A represents a bead of one colour of a given pair, and B a bead of the other colour) was as follows:

Condition 1: A A A B A A A A A B B A A A A A A A A B
Condition 2: A A A B A A A A B A B B B A B B B B A B

Belief maintenance/change, as well as formation, was investigated in Condition 2. It will be seen that, in this condition, the first 10 draws support the hypothesis that the beads are being drawn from the jar with the predominantly A coloured beads, but the final 10 beads are inconsistent with this hypothesis, favouring the alternative.

The administration of the Synonyms part of the Mill Hill Vocabularly Scale (Raven 1982) was followed by the experimental tasks. Before beginning each condition, subjects were asked to read the relevant instructions. These explained that the jars contained beads in the proportion 85:15. The instructions were clarified with the subject, who then practised use of the response board. Emphasis was placed on the same points as specified in the pilot study, concerning sampling with replacement in the same jar, and that, for Condition 1, subjects were allowed as many trials as they needed to be completely sure as to which jar was chosen. In Condition 1 the trial was stopped when the subject indicated which jar had been chosen. The experimenter then asked the subject, 'Are you completely certain which jar has been chosen?'. If the subject indicated any uncertainty, additional draws were offered until the subject indicated that s/he had decided with certainty. In Condition 2 all subjects were shown 20 draws and were asked after each draw to indicate their estimate of the likelihood of jar A having been chosen.

There were two experimental conditions, each combining two conditions from the pilot study:

Condition 1: A YES–NO response mode was used in this condition. Subjects were shown beads drawn from one (hidden) jar in a predetermined sequence. They were asked whether or not they required more draws before they came to a decision as to which jar had been chosen by pointing to one of two cards bearing the message 'More items please' or 'No more items, I have decided'. When the subjects pointed to the stop card, they were asked which jar they thought the draw/draws came from. In addition, before the first draw, subjects were required to estimate the probability of a particular colour bead being drawn. Once subjects reached a decision, the trial was terminated.

Condition 2: A probabilistic response mode was used in this condition. Twenty draws of beads from one (hidden) jar were shown in a predetermined sequence. After each draw, subjects indicated the relative probabilities that they attached to the draw having come from either of the two jars, using the response board. In this condition the trial was not terminated when the subject expressed complete certainty that one particular jar had been chosen, but continued for 20 draws for all subjects.

Dependent variables

Condition 1

1. *Draws to decision*. The number of draws taken to reach a decision.

2. *Initial certainty*. The prior estimate of the likelihood of a particular colour bead being chosen on the very first draw. The normative

(Bayesian) estimate is 50 per cent; scores above 50 therefore represent over-confident estimates. (In Huq *et al.* this variable is referred to as 'event estimation'.)

3. *Errors in decision-making* (jar A being considered correct).

Condition 2

4. *Initial posterior estimate.* The first estimate of the likelihood of jar A having been chosen after being presented with the first draw, calculated as the actual estimate made. (The Bayesian estimate is 85 per cent; scores above 85 represent over-confidence and below 85 represent under-confidence.)

5. *Draws to certainty* that jar A has been chosen, calculated as the number of draws to an estimate of 100 per cent or, where 100 per cent is not reached, 85 per cent estimated for two draws.

6a. *The effect of confirmatory evidence on judgement.* The effect of confirmatory evidence on a subsequent estimate, calculated as the second posterior estimate minus the first posterior estimate. (A positive score shows an increase in confidence following confirmatory evidence.)

6b. *The effect of disconfirmatory evidence on judgement.* The effect of potentially disconfirmatory evidence on a subsequent estimate calculated as the posterior estimate 3 (after three pink beads) minus posterior estimate 4, after the first green bead. (A positive score shows a decrease in confidence following potentially disconfirmatory evidence.)

7. *Errors in decision-making,* after the first 10 draws. The correct decision is taken to be a probability estimate of greater than 85 per cent favouring jar A.

8. *Draws from draw 10 to a change in estimate.* The number of items to a change in the estimate, having already reached a decision, calculated as the number of draws from draw 10 to any change.

9. *The size of the first estimate change,* calculated as the difference between the size of the estimate at draw 10 and the estimate at the first point of change.

10. *Final decision.* The final decision after the last draw, with respect to the probability that jar A had been chosen.

Subjects

Subjects were in four groups, two groups of deluded subjects and two control groups. The deluded subjects were selected according to the following criteria:

1. Abnormal beliefs satisfying the DSM-III (American Psychiatric Association 1980) criteria for delusions.

2. Current delusions expressed in interview (see Chapter 8) at a high level of conviction.

3. *Either* current symptoms satisfying the Research Diagnostic Criteria for Schizophrenia (Spitzer *et al.* 1978) *or* the DSM III-R criteria for delusional disorder (paranoia) (American Psychiatric Association 1987) as assessed by a research psychiatrist (S Wessely).

4. Aged 18 to 65 years.

Thirteen subjects (three women, ten men) satisfied these criteria for a diagnosis of schizophrenia (S) and 14 (four women, ten men) for a diagnosis of delusional disorder (P). Because subjects with a diagnosis of paranoia are rare, subjects were sought not only at a psychiatric but also at a special hospital. Schizophrenic subjects were also taken from both the special hospital and the psychiatric hosptial. Patients from the general psychiatric hospital were both in-patients and out-patients. All but four of the deluded subjects were currently being prescribed anti-psychotic medication.

A normal control group (N) of four women and nine men, totalling 13, consisted of individuals aged between 18 and 65 years with no history of psychiatric treatment, drawn largely from hospital nursing, ancillary, and clerical staff. An anxious control group (A) consisted of 14 subjects (four women, ten men) currently receiving treatment for generalized anxiety disorder, agoraphobia, or a specific phobia, and aged between 18 and 65 years. Of this group, six were receiving medication (five subjects minor tranquillizers and one subject anti-depressant medication). Anxious patients were chosen because they are not known to show a reasoning bias on this task (in contrast to obsessionals), and generally have no history of delusions. (A check was made for each patient that this latter point was true.) An effort was made to enlist anxious subjects with relatively severe disorders by including in-patients, and five of the group were currently receiving in-patient care, although the duration of stay was very much less than the deluded subjects'.

All subjects completed the Mill Hill Vocabulary Scale (synonyms). For all groups, any scoring below the tenth percentile were excluded; a total of three were excluded for this reason, one subject from each of the schizophrenic, paranoid, and anxious control groups. Two patients at the special hospital, thought to be suitable for inclusion in the study, refused to take part. The case note data indicate that one would have been diagnosed as schizophrenic and the other as paranoid. Subjects were told that they were being invited to take part in a test of the way people reason and, for those who were patients, that the outcome would have no bearing on their psychiatric care. Subjects' characteristics are presented in Table 7.2.

Analysis of variance revealed no significant differences between the groups for either age or Mill Hill vocabulary score. Length of contact with psychiatric services and total duration of in-patient care are given in Table 7.3. Current patient status is also given. The anxious control group had shorter contact and less in-patient care than the other groups. All of the schizophrenic subjects were in-patients as were 10 of the paranoid subjects. Similar numbers of the schizophrenic (8) and the paranoid groups (6) were in-patients at a special hospital.

Results

Because of the large variance in response, particularly in the schizophrenic group, a non-parametric analysis of variance was employed, the Kruskal–Wallis test. As the pilot study's results

Table 7.2 *Subject characteristics*

Group		N	Sex		Age (years)		Mill Hill Vocabulary score	
			F	M	Mean	SD	Mean	SD
Schizophrenia	(S)	13	3	10	37.5	13.6	27.0	3.0
Paranoia/ delusional disorder	(P)	14	4	10	41.2	12.1	27.2	3.5
Anxious control	(A)	14	4	10	36.7	14.1	28.5	3.6
Normal control	(N)	13	4	9	42.5	12.8	26.8	5.2
Significance		—	NS		NS		NS	

NS = not significant.

Table 7.3 *Contact with psychiatric services*

Group	Years of psychiatric contact		Total months in-patient care		Current patient status	
	Mean	SD	Mean	SD	In-patient	Out-patient
Schizo-phrenia (S)	14.3	11.5	72.1	92.6	13	0
Paranoia/delusional disorder (D)	15.1	13.1	49.0	91.5	10	4
Anxious control (A)	4.9	6.1	2.0	3.5	5	9
Significance	F 3.9, d.f.=2 $p<0.05$		NS $(p=0.06)$		$\chi^2=12.9$, d.f.=2 $p=<0.001$	

NS = not significant.

indicated that the deluded subjects were more likely to give 'extreme' responses (such as very rapid decision-making and large probability estimates), for certain variables, scores were categorized into 'extreme' versus 'not extreme' (see Garety 1990 for details) and a separate chi-square analysis was conducted to compare deluded with control subjects.

In Condition 1, in which the formation of beliefs was studied, a significant difference between the groups was found for draws to decision (Kruskal–Wallis $\chi^2=11.85$, d.f. 3, $p<0.01$). The results are presented in Table 7.4. and graphically in Fig. 7.1. The results for Condition 2 are presented in Table 7.5.

The schizophrenic and paranoid groups requested fewer items of information before reaching a decision. Post hoc paired comparisons were carried out using the Mann–Whitney U Test. On no variable were there statistically significant differences between the two deluded groups. For the variable 'draws to decision', there was a significant difference between the schizophrenic and normal control groups ($p<0.005$) and a trend to statistically significant differences (applying the Bonferroni criterion (Fleiss 1986)) between the schizophrenic and anxious control groups ($p<0.03$) and between the paranoid and normal groups ($p<0.02$).

With respect to extreme patterns of responding, 11 deluded subjects (S = 7, P = 4) reached a decision after only *one* item of information,

Table 7.4. *Mean scores on dependent variables for the four groups, Condition 1*

Groups	1. Draws to decision		2. Initial certainty		3. Errors
	Mean	SD	Mean	SD	
S	2.38	1.94	60.9	22.5	2
P	3.00	2.29	66.7	19.5	2
A	3.71	1.68	66.5	16.8	0
N	5.38	3.15	56.3	26.6	0
Kruskal–Wallis χ^2 (d.f. 3)	11.85		1.5		0.87
Significance	$p < 0.01$		NS		NS

NS = not significant.

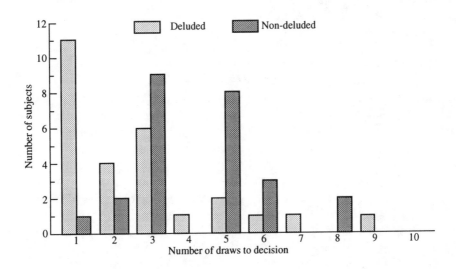

Fig. 7.1 Draws to decision—task 1.

Table 7.5 *Mean scores on dependent variables for the four groups, Condition 2*

Groups	4. Initial posterior estimate		5. Draws to certainty		6a. Effect of evidence on judgement (confirmatory)		6b. Effect of evidence on judgement (disconfirmatory)		7. Errors	8. Draws to change		9. Size of change	
	Mean	SD	Mean	SD	Mean	SD	Mean	SD		Mean	SD	Mean	SD
S	62.9	32.0	4.4	2.8	10.1	47.9	11.2	49.3	2	2.2	1.3	40.5	39.1
P	73.6	20.8	3.3	2.0	10.1	14.8	9.1	15.1	0	3.7	2.2	29.6	30.6
A	71.6	13.9	3.9	1.7	9.1	5.2	0.1	14.1	0	4.2	2.6	15.8	10.6
N	57.1	22.9	5.4	1.8	9.1	23.7	4.3	12.0	0	4.1	2.6	26.5	25.0
Kruskal – Wallis χ^2 (d.f. 3)	3.8		5.8		1.7		9.03			5.8		2.7	
Significance	NS		NS		NS		$p<0.05$		NS	NS		NS	

NS = not significant.

Schizophrenic and paranoid groups

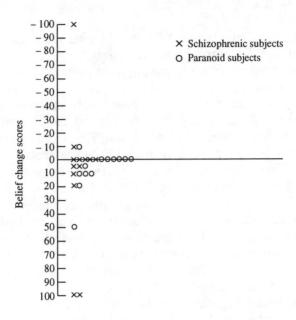

Anxious and normal groups

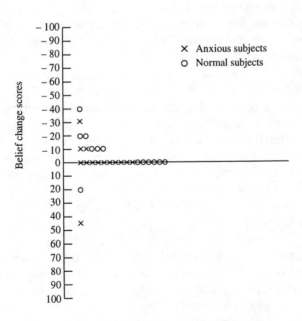

Fig. 7.2 Effect of evidence on judgement—task 2.

compared with only one (normal) control subject ($\chi^2 = 8.7$, d.f. 1, $p < 0.005$) (see Fig. 7.1).

There were no significant differences between the groups on the other Condition 1 variable, initial certainty.

Very few errors in decision-making were made. In Condition 1 two schizophrenic subjects and two paranoid subjects made errors and in Condition 2 two (different) schizophrenic subjects made errors.

In Condition 2, in which the processes of belief formation and maintenance/change were studied, a significant difference between the groups was found with respect to the subjects' response to potentially disconfirmatory evidence (variable 6b, Kruskal−Wallis $\chi^2 = 9.03$, d.f. 3, $p < 0.05$) (see Table 7.5 and Fig. 7.2). Mann−Whitney U Tests between pairs of groups revealed no significant differences between the two deluded groups on this variable. The schizophrenic and paranoid subjects were more likely to respond to one item of potentially disconfirmatory evidence by revising their estimates downwards, while the anxious and normal groups were more likely to make either no change in estimate or to continue to affirm their initial hypothesis by increasing their estimates slightly. Four deluded subjects (S=3, P=1) made estimate changes of more than 50 per cent, compared with no estimate changes of that magnitude in the control groups.

There were no significant differences in overall group performance between groups on the other variables. There were also no significant differences, using the Mann−Whitney U Test, between the two deluded groups on any of the variables.

With respect to extreme responses the combined deluded groups showed a higher frequency of such responses on four of the remaining variables, although these largely failed to reach statistical significance. On draws to certainty, five deluded subjects decided on the hypothesis after the very first draw, and only one (normal) control; on initial posterior estimate, six deluded subjects estimated at 95 per cent or over on the basis of one draw, compared with two controls (A = 1, N = 1); on number of draws to change in estimate, after certainty was reached, six deluded subjects and only one (anxious) control made a change at the first potentially disconfirmatory draw, a marginally statistically significant difference ($\chi^2 = 4.5$, d.f. 1, $p < 0.05$, before Yates' correction; $\chi^2 = 3.0$, d.f. 1, $p = 0.08$ with Yates' correction); with respect to the size of this change of estimate, five deluded subjects made a change of greater than 65 per cent, compared with one non-deluded (N) subject.

The data were also analysed to investigate whether there were any symptomatic or demographic differences between the extreme responders and the other subjects. The deluded subjects were divided into those who made a decision after one draw on Condition 1 (N = 11) and those who requested more items of information (N = 16). There were no differences on any demographic characteristics (age, sex, length of current in-patient admission, years from first psychiatric contact, and total months in-patient care). However, the extreme responders did score significantly lower on the Mill Hill Vocabulary Test (mean 25.5, SD 1.8) than the other deluded subjects (mean 28.2, SD 3.5) $t = 2.3$, d.f. 26 ($p < 0.05$).

Information was also collected about the current mental state of subjects (see Chapter 8 for full details), and comparisons were made between extreme responders and the rest in terms of these variables. Extreme responders were more likely to express high conviction about their own delusional beliefs, when measured in terms of any possible doubts ($\chi^2 = 6.17$, d.f. 1, $p < 0.01$), and were also more likely to be experiencing or noticing, within the past week, anomalous events which led them to believe their delusions (for example auditory hallucinations) ($\chi^2 = 6.2$, d.f. 2, $p < 0.05$).

Discussion

The results of the study confirm the principal finding of the pilot study (Huq *et al.* 1988) that deluded subjects request less information before reaching a decision on a probabilistic inference task than either non-deluded psychiatric or normal controls. A substantial number (41 per cent in this study, compared with 47 per cent in Huq *et al.*) of the deluded subjects reached a decision after only *one* item of information was presented, at the objective probability level of 85 per cent. Although, overall, the deluded groups appear better (more Bayesian) reasoners with respect to hypothesis formation than controls, who are on average over-cautious, averaging the scores obscures a tendency to hasty decision-making in some members of the experimental groups.

With respect to sub-groups within the deluded sample, biases in reasoning did not follow clear diagnostic divisions. It was noted that Chapman and Chapman (1988) regard reasoning abnormalities as more likely to be present in schizophrenic subjects, while a hypothesis that delusions are normal accounts of abnormal experiences might imply that subjects in whom anomalous experiences are less evident, such as subjects with delusional disorder, would be more likely to show abnormalities of reasoning. However, the style of reasoning identified here was present in members of both groups, and in this sample is more common (although not significant statistically) in

patients diagnosed schizophrenic: seven (45 per cent) of the schizophrenics responded with a decision after one draw and four (29 per
cent) of those with delusional disorder.

The other finding of Huq *et al.*, that deluded subjects express
higher levels of certainty after the first item of information is
presented, was not replicated, although it is of note that six deluded
subjects (compared with two controls) made estimates after the first
draw of 95 per cent or over, when the objective (Bayesian) probability
is 85 per cent.

The findings which bear on belief maintenance/change are interesting. They do not suggest that deluded subjects are characteristically incorrigible. The schizophrenic and paranoid groups showed
a greater, rather than lesser, inclination to reduce their confidence in
their estimates in the face of potentially contradictory evidence than
controls. Three of the schizophrenic group completely changed their
estimates to 100 per cent certainty in the *opposite* direction. Here
some members of the deluded groups are not clinging tenaciously to
their hypotheses, but rapidly changing them. This is consistent with
studies of information processing cited in Chapter 3 which emphasize
the greater influence accorded by schizophrenics to the immediate
environmental stimuli than to the effects of prior learning (Salzinger
1984; Hemsley 1987; Gray *et al.* 1991a). It may also be relevant to
Chapman and Chapman's view of a selection bias in schizophrenic
subjects with respect to focusing on prominent and neglecting weaker
stimuli compared with normals.

The responses on the other variables are consistent with this,
although the results generally fail to reach statistical significance: the
deluded (particularly the schizophrenic) subjects show a trend to
changing their estimates (variable 8) very rapidly once certainty has
been reached; furthermore, this immediate response is not a cautious
one — the size of the estimate change (variable 9) also shows a trend
to being large (over 65 per cent) so that these subjects actually adjust,
on the basis of one item of information, to favouring the contradictory
hypothesis. Perhaps most tellingly, when the final decision is
scrutinized, the deluded subjects do not show a tendency to hold
tenaciously to their initial hypothesis. Only six deluded subjects
(S = 4, P = 2) strongly favoured jar A at the end, compared with
nine controls (A = 4, N = 5).

A substantial proportion of the deluded subjects therefore formed
strong hypotheses more readily, but a significant minority were also
more ready to revise them: over-confidence and extreme judgements
appear more characteristic than incorrigibility.

However, as in the Huq *et al.* study, extreme responses were present in only a sub-group of the deluded subjects. One-half to two-thirds of the deluded subjects responded normally. Variation in responses in schizophrenic subjects has been found in many other studies (for example Colbourn and Lishman 1979; David 1987). David, in a study of colour naming and matching, found that schizophrenics who demonstrated a critical pattern of errors were more likely to show first-rank symptoms and showed less cerebral atrophy. The present findings suggest that the 'extreme' responders may be of lower verbal intelligence, more convinced of their delusions, and more likely to be currently subject to anomalous experiences.

CONCLUSIONS

The results of this study add to the growing body of evidence for judgemental biases in deluded subjects. These findings suggest that a 'jumping to conclusions' bias applies not only to delusion-relevant material or to perceptions, but also to a neutral content task. The Bayesian model of probabilistic reasoning, and the Edwards task derived from it and used in a modified form here, have provided a valuable normative framework within which subjects' performance can be evaluated.

The judgemental bias was not confined to one diagnostic category, whether schizophrenic or paranoid, although there are some indications that it may be more common in patients diagnosed as schizophrenic. Whether or not this proves to be the case, it is clear that the bias found in the pilot study and the present one occurs in only a sub-group of deluded subjects, and it is clearly of great interest to identify any distinguishing characteristics. One intriguing association in these data is between the judgemental bias and perceptual anomalies; could both possibly result from a common cause? These issues will be considered in more detail in the final chapter.

In this study attention was paid to the maintenance of hypotheses as well as their formation. The deluded subjects again showed a judgemental bias, but the bias was paradoxically one which facilitated the abandonment of their hypotheses (and the formation of new ones) rather than incorrigible maintenance. This would suggest that the phenomenon of delusional incorrigibility may not itself result from a reasoning abnormality, but represents a normal manifestation of tenacity for important and strongly held beliefs.

In the light of these findings, it may prove instructive to return to the experiences of the deluded people themselves. What accounts do they give of the formation and maintenance of their beliefs? It is this which is addressed next.

8 Reasoning about delusions

INTRODUCTION

In Chapter 6, theories of delusion formation were discussed. A number of processes are thought, by different theorists, to be implicated in the formation (and maintenance) of delusions, including abnormal perceptual experience, abnormal mood, and abnormal reasoning. It was argued that the reasoning of deluded individuals should be studied to investigate judgemental biases in processing neutral material and the resulting study is described in Chapter 7. However, there have also been remarkably few systematic studies of the way that deluded people reason about their own delusions; much of the theorizing derives from anecdotal case reports.

In this chapter, therefore, we describe a study* in which we examined deluded people's own accounts of their delusions, in terms of the reasons they give for forming and maintaining their beliefs. The same problem of setting a norm for reasoning discussed in Chapter 6 applies, and we propose the same solution. A Bayesian framework can be used to evaluate deluded subjects' delusional belief formation and maintenance. As noted above, Fischhoff and Beyth-Marom (1983) describe a number of stages at which an individual, in forming or maintaining a belief, can deviate from the norm: these include the nature of the hypothesis (for example is the belief testable?), the assessment by the individual of the strength of the belief, the extent to which that assessment is consistent with the strength of the negation of the belief, and the way in which the individual evaluates new information.

In this chapter the development and administration of a structured interview, using a Bayesian framework, to study the reasoning of deluded subjects about their delusions is described. Also considered are the extent to which deluded subjects report that perceptual experiences and mood states are involved at the stages of belief

---

*The interview described in this study has subsequently been incorporated in modified form in the MADS (Maudsley Assessment of Delusions Schedule): Buchanan *et al.* (1993). *Br. J. Psychiat.*, **163**, 77–81.

formation and maintenance. It was noted in Chapter 1 that people may not be able to report accurately on their thinking processes (Nisbett and Wilson 1977); clearly this limitation may apply here. What is being studied are the accounts that subjects give, rather than the actual processes themselves. A further difficulty here is that the accounts concern events in the past. The accuracy of such retrospective reports may be imperfect.

It is likely that different processes are involved in the formation of different types of delusions. In this study, as in the one reported in Chapter 7, and for the same reasons, the investigation was restricted to subjects who do not have a primary affective disorder or known organic pathology. The study was confined to a comparison of subjects with a clear diagnosis of schizophrenia with those diagnosed as suffering from delusional disorder (paranoia).

The aims of the study were:

(1) to develop a structured interview to detail deluded subjects' accounts of the formation and maintenance of their delusional beliefs, employing a Bayesian framework;

(2) to assess the inter-rater reliability of the interview;

(3) to assess the extent to which deluded subjects report anomalous perceptual experiences and abnormal mood states as involved in the belief formation/maintenance;

(4) to categorize the content of the delusional belief statements, and to assess the reliability of this categorization and of ratings of their bizarreness; and,

(5) to compare patients with diagnoses of schizophrenia and delusional disorder with respect to their responses.

THE REASONING ABOUT DELUSIONS STRUCTURED INTERVIEW STUDY

Method

Subjects

This study employed the same subjects as the study reported in Chapter 7, except that three additional patients were interviewed, two with a diagnosis of schizophrenia (S) and one with a diagnosis of paranoia (P). One subject in the paranoid group in the previous study was not included because he refused to complete the interview. There were therefore a total of 29 subjects, 15 with a diagnosis of schizophrenia and 14 with a diagnosis of paranoia. The diagnostic criteria and assessment of current delusions were as given in Chapter 7. Fourteen of the patients in the schizophrenic group were in-patients, and one was a day patient, and four of the paranoid group were out-patients, the rest being in-patients. Similar numbers of the groups (S = 8) and (P = 7) were in-patients at a special hospital. Subjects' characteristics are given in Table 8.1. There were no significant differences between the groups in gender, age, contact with psychiatric services, or Mill Hill Vocabulary score.

The interview

The interview was designed to consider the stages of belief formation and maintenance as specified by Fischhoff and Beyth-Marom (1983), (and described above). The full interview, together with explanatory notes for interviewers, is given in Appendices 1 and 2.

After first identifying the belief to be studied, an assessment of the conviction with which the belief is held follows, employing an assessment both of the probability of the hypothesis, $p(H)$, and the probability of the negation of the hypothesis, $p(not-H)$.

The way in which the belief started is then considered, in terms of suddenness/gradualness and whether it had the quality of a worry or a realization/thinking about the possibility.

The data on which the hypothesis was originally based are then discussed, with particular reference to whether they were data *internal* to the subject or *external*. By internal is meant a mood state, a perceptual experience for which no external source can be clearly identified or some other state internal to the subject, which others are not apparently experiencing. External data are events capable of being witnessed by people other than the subject (even if they have not in fact been). The type of internal or external state/event is specified.

Factors which are reported by the subject to be maintaining the belief at present, apart from the initial stated cause, are then explored. These are also categorized as internal/external and subtypes. Whether there have been any events or experiences in the current week is also noted.

The search for information is considered next. Does the subject describe seeking any evidence either to confirm/prove the correctness of his/her view, or, on the contrary, to test whether the view may be mistaken? If there is information search, a check is made on the information value of the datum: is the information confirmatory, disconfirmatory, or apparently irrelevant?

Table 8.1 *Subjects' characteristics*

Group	N	Gender	Age		Years contact with Psychiatric Services		Total months in-patient care		Mill Hill Vocabulary score	
			Mean	SD	Mean	SD	Mean	SD	Mean	SD
Schizophrenic (S)	15	F = 3, M = 12	42.3	16.0	17.4	13.2	89.5	134.4	25.2	4.17
Paranoid (P)	14	F = 4, M = 10	43.6	12.8	15.6	12.6	57.0	90.7	27.3	3.6
Significance	NS	NS	NS		NS		NS		NS	

NS = not significant.

In the light of any evidence cited, how does this affect the probability of the hypothesis, $p(H/D)$? Also, what is the probability of the negation of the hypothesis, even given the truth of the datum, $p(\text{not-}H/D)$? A check is then made on whether the discussion has cast any doubt in the subject's mind on the certainty of the belief.

It is clearly not always possible within the constraints of an interview to find actual contradictory evidence concerning a subject's delusional belief, in order to evaluate how new data are assessed. (It may also not always be desirable with certain patients who appear very distressed.) However, it is generally possible (and less threatening) to devise a hypothetical contradiction to test the subject's response to evidential challenges to the belief (even if hypothetical). Brett-Jones *et al.* (1987) devised a measure, called Reaction to Hypothetical Contradiction (RTHC), for this purpose (described in full in Chapter 4). Subjects are presented with a hypothetical but plausible piece of evidence which is contradictory to their belief, and are asked how this would affect their belief. The reply is categorized into one of four possible responses.

Finally, subjects are asked about action which is a direct consequence of their belief. Not included are coming into hospital or changes in routine consequent on this unless this was volitional and a direct consequence of the belief. The responses to this question are only coded if the behaviour change is verified by direct observation, or information from staff or the case notes.

Content of delusions categorization

In Chapter 5, in which a study of the characteristics of delusions was reported, the beliefs were categorized using a modification of Forgus and De Wolfe's (1974) categories. In the present study the same categorization was again employed, although an additional (sixth) category, concerning interference with thinking processes, was added.

The categories were:

(1) positive self, for example 'I am Jesus Christ';

(2) positive world, for example 'The world is being purified through an invisible fire';

(3) negative self, for example 'I am dementing';

(4) negative world, for example 'The world will end this month';

(5) paranoid, for example 'The Mafia are plotting to kill me';

(6) thought interference (broadcasting, insertion, control), for example 'A micro-computer is reading my mind'.

It has been noted that delusions are thought to be remarkable for their bizarreness and inherent implausibility (Jaspers 1913; Mullen 1979). In addition to categorizing content, raters were asked to rate the bizarreness and inherent implausibility of the belief statements.

Procedure

There were two interviewers, P.A.G. and a psychiatrist, Dr S Wessely. They each conducted approximately half of the interviews and coded the responses of the other subjects' taped interviews for assessments of inter-rater reliability. S.W. also made the diagnoses of schizophrenia or delusional disorder, according to the criteria specified in Chapter 7.

Standard demographic data were collected from the case notes and the psychiatrist responsible for the patient's care was asked to complete a form with seven questions about current mental state.

RESULTS

Inter-rater reliability of interview responses

A full list of subjects' belief statements is given in Appendix 3. The inter-rater reliability of subjects' responses was calculated using the kappa statistic (Cohen 1960) (Table 8.2). For 15 items, kappas of 0.78–1.00 were achieved, all at least $p < 0.0002$. The remaining four items were $x = 0.56–0.70$, $p < 0.005$. The coding of the items was therefore highly reliable.

Interview responses, and comparisons between the schizophrenic and paranoid groups

1. Conviction

Both groups expressed high conviction, 67 per cent S and 64 per cent P absolute certainty. On a five-point scale (1–5), the mean conviction score was 4.3 SD 1.1, with no difference between the groups.

2. Inverse conviction (probability of not-H)

When expressed in terms of the probability of the negation of the hypothesis, in both groups a small number of subjects gave responses

Table 8.2 *Reasoning about delusions structured interview: inter-rater reliabilities of responses*

Item		x	p
1.	Conviction	1.000	<0.00001
2.	Inverse conviction	0.96	<0.00001
3.	Start	0.93	<0.00001
4.	Internal state	0.81	<0.0001
5.	Type of internal state	0.78	<0.00001
6.	External event	0.79	<0.0002
7.	Type of external event	0.70	<0.0005
8.	More recent state/event	0.92	<0.00001
9.	Recent internal state	0.89	<0.00005
10.	Type of recent internal state	0.92	<0.00001
11.	Recent external event	0.67	<0.005
12.	Type of recent external event	0.56	<0.001
13.	Information search	1.000	<0.00001
14.	Type of information	0.91	<0.00001
15.	Conviction given data	0.92	<0.00001
16.	Probability of not-H, given data	1.000	<0.00001
17.	Possibly mistaken	1.000	<0.00001
18.	Reaction to hypothetical contradiction	0.57	<0.0005
19.	Action	0.91	<0.00005

which admitted of more doubt than their estimates of $p(H)$ should allow, that is $p(H) + p(\text{not-H}) > 1$. Thus, only 60 per cent S and 50 per cent P expressed no possibility of the truth of not-H. However, the conviction score was highly correlated (Pearson product moment) with inverse conviction ($r = 0.92$, $p < 0.0001$).

3. Start

In both groups, approximately one-third of subjects described their beliefs as starting suddenly (33 per cent S, 36 per cent P); however, 50 per cent of the paranoid group described the start as a gradual worry, while 40 per cent of the schizophrenic group described a gradual entertaining of the hypothesis. A chi-square test for differences between the two groups yields $\chi^2 = 9.48$, d.f. 3, $p < 0.05$. However, there are more than 20 per cent of cells with an expected frequency of less than five, violating the requirements for a valid chi-square.

4. Internal state at start

Eighty per cent of the S group, and 64 per cent of the P group describe their beliefs as caused by an internal state.

5. Type of internal state

Only three subjects (S = 2, P = 1) described a mood state. Twelve subjects (S = 8, P = 4) reported a clear abnormal perceptual experience, most commonly auditory in the S group, although only one P subject reported an auditory phenomenon. Three P subjects reported 'smells'. A number of the internal states were less clearly perceptual. These were: puzzlement (S), odd thoughts and an awareness of evil (S), mental and physical changes (P), memory of being hypnotized (P), pain and pins and needles (P), and itching (P).

6. External event

Seven S subjects and ten P subjects reported noticing some event external to them which caused them to believe their delusion. For three S and five P subjects the external events apparently occurred in the absence of internal states, while for the others both categories were regarded as causative. Examples of external events reported by the subjects are: horses running in a race with special names, such as 'King David' (the patient's name being David), the GP changing the tablets of the patient's mother (the belief that the GP was trying to kill the mother), and a newspaper article about tax evaders (the belief that the Inland Revenue are keeping him under surveillance).

7. Type of external event

All events were coded as observable.

8. Recent states or events

All subjects bar one (P) reported some event or state since the initial formation of the belief which had led them to continue to believe it. Sixty per cent of the S and 50 per cent of the P group reported events/states in the past week.

9. Recent internal state

Eleven S (73 per cent) and ten P (71 per cent) subjects reported a recent internal state.

10. Type of recent internal state

Two subjects in each group reported abnormal mood states. Clear perceptual experiences were reported by eight S and five P subjects. Less clearly categorizable internal states were reported by one S and three P subjects.

11. Recent external event

Similar numbers of subjects who reported noticing events around them at the beginning reported them as occurring more recently (S = 8, P = 10). These include noticing significant numbers, or overhearing comments thought to be directed at the subject, for example 'don't you dare say anything to her'.

12. Type of recent external event

These are all coded as observable, bar two in the S group, coded as not potentially observable.

13. Information search

Approximately half of the S group (7) and only two of the P group reported no information search, $\chi^2 = 3.55$, d.f. 1, $p = 0.06$. (More than 20 per cent of cells with an expected frequency of less than five.) There is a trend towards P subjects being more likely to seek out information or evidence concerning their belief.

14. Type of information

All 12 of the P subjects who sought evidence, reported seeking confirmatory information, while four S subjects reported the same. One S subject reported seeking apparently irrelevant information, $\chi^2 = 10.2$, d.f. 1, $p < 0.001$. (More than 20 per cent of cells with an expected frequency of less than five.)

15. Conviction in the light of the data

Four of the S subjects could offer no evidence, whether internal or external. Of those subjects who did offer data, only one subject in each group expressed clear doubts about the belief in the light of it. All of the other subjects were certain or almost certain.

(Mean conviction score 4.66, compared with mean score of 4.3 at the beginning of the interview.)

16. Probability of not-H, given D

Seventy per cent of the S group (who offered data) and 64 per cent of the P group believed that their data proved the truth of the belief, that is the belief could not be false, given the data. Only three subjects (S = 1, P = 2) admitted a significant possibility that the data did not necessarily imply the truth of the hypothesis. For example, one subject who believed he was being 'set up by the CIA and used as a guinea pig' gave as evidence for this the fact that he had been 'treated badly' by the Veterans Administration and the FBI (for example letters of complaint not replied to). He accepted that it was quite possible that these bureaucracies often treat people badly. He said 'yes, perhaps I was treated just like any other guy'.

17. Is there any possibility of being mistaken?

Five subjects (S = 2, P = 3) thought there was some possibility of being mistaken.

18. Reaction to hypothetical contradiction

Only one (S) subject's belief appeared untestable hypothetically. Sixteen subjects (S = 8, P = 8) ignored or rejected the relevance of the counter-instance. Seven subjects (S = 4, P = 3) accommodated the counter-instance into their belief system. Two (S = 1, P = 1) thought they would reduce their conviction levels, and two (S = 1, P = 1) thought they would dismiss their beliefs, if faced with such evidence.

19. Action

One-third of the S group and 86 per cent of the P group reported acting on their beliefs (independently verified). This is a statistically significant difference between the groups: $\chi^2 = 8.19$, d.f. 1, $p < 0.005$.

Content, bizarreness, and implausibility ratings

Categorization of content was assessed for reliability, using three raters — the two interviewers and a psychologist. The mean kappa was 0.77 (SD 0.13), $p < 0.00001$.

Although the number of cells, and the size of the sample again yielded too many cells with an expected frequency of less than five, the chi-square is indicative of a difference between the groups for belief content ($x^2 = 18.63$, d.f. 4, $p < 0.001$). For the schizophrenic group six subjects had 'positive self' beliefs, six 'thought interference', and one each negative self, negative world, and paranoid. In the paranoid group seven subjects had 'negative self' beliefs, six paranoid, and one 'positive self'.

The bizarreness and inherent implausibility of the belief statements were rated by three psychologists, including the first author. The mean weighted kappa for bizarreness was 0.31 (SD 0.23), $p < 0.05$. Mean weighted kappa for inherent implausibility was 0.40 (SD 0.11), $p < 0.01$. The ratings between bizarreness and implausibility were highly correlated, for example $r = 0.84$, $p < 0.0001$, rater A. Bizarreness and implausibility were rated on a seven-point scale (1–7). For each rater, the mean bizarreness and implausibility ratings were significantly higher for the statements of the schizophrenic group than for the paranoid group. For example, rater A's scores were:

Bizarreness S = $\bar{x}$ 5.5, P = $\bar{x}$ 2.6, t 5.45, d.f. 27, $p < 0.0001$

and

Implausibility S = $\bar{x}$ 5.7, P = $\bar{x}$ 3.9, t 2.47, d.f. 27, $p < 0.05$.

Demographic and current mental state data

There were very few differences between the groups in terms of demographic and mental state data. There were no differences in terms of case-note records of marital status (S = 2, P = 4 married), employment (S = 2, P = 5 employed), types of medication, criminal convictions (50 per cent of both groups), or a history of violence (again approximately 50 per cent of both groups).

Consistent with the interview finding, more subjects in the paranoid group than in the schizophrenic group were recorded as acting on their beliefs, both currently (S = 4, P = 9) or at some point in the past. Whereas five schizophrenic subjects were thought never to have acted on the beliefs, this was true of no paranoid subjects. ($x^2 = 7.0$, d.f. 2, $p < 0.05$, although again more than 20 per cent of the cells had an expected frequency of less than five.)

In terms of mental state data, no paranoid subjects were thought by their psychiatrist to experience auditory hallucinations, while 70 per cent of the schizophrenic group were thought to do so ($x^2 = 13.8$, d.f. 1, $p < 0.0005$). There was a non-significant trend for the paranoid subjects to be more likely to be regarded as depressed (S = 0, P = 4). There was also a non-significant trend for the paranoid subjects to show a poorer response to medication (no response S = 1, P = 7), and for the delusions to be thought more stable (stable S = 4, P = 9).

DISCUSSION

The interview revealed that deluded subjects are able to provide understandable accounts of the development and continuance of their delusional beliefs.

The Bayesian framework provided a useful structure for discussing the stages of belief formation and maintenance, and for considering the nature of the information cited by interviewees as causally responsible for their beliefs. However, it may of course be that subjects misrepresented the reasons for belief formation or maintenance, either deliberately or for other reasons such as not having access to the processes or imperfect memory.

Recruiting subjects from a special hospital is likely to have biased the results. Such patients could only be released on the recommendation of their doctors, and were also, for the most part, convicted of serious crimes for which their mental state was thought to be responsible. Subjects were assured that the interviews would not be communicated to the hospital staff, and appeared in general to believe this. In this context, it was striking how many subjects related their beliefs concerning, for example, their persecution and the subsequent steps (for example murder) that they took, without any hint of an apology. The number of subjects with a history of violence, and perhaps of acting on their beliefs, is inflated by this means of subject selection when compared with a normal mental hospital population. However, in terms of comparisons between diagnostic groups, care was taken to ensure that similar numbers of subjects in each group were drawn from this setting.

One purpose of the interview was to investigate the role of abnormal perceptual experience and abnormal mood state in the formation and maintenance of delusions in groups of psychotic patients without a primary affective disorder or known organic pathology, and to assess style of reasoning. The study has yielded some interesting findings.

The initial statement of conviction, which on average is very high, is predictable. When subjects are asked about the probability of the negation of their hypothesis, three subjects violate the normative rule that $p(H) + p(\text{not-H}) = 1$, by expressing both certainty and a possibility that they are mistaken.

An attempt was made to distinguish beliefs which started suddenly and those which developed gradually. One-third described a sudden start, although none was clearly of the Jasperian 'primary' delusion type in the sense of the sudden apprehension of meaning from an unexceptional 'correct' perception. For the rest, in whom the development was described as gradual, those in the schizophrenic group 'entertained the possibility' while those in the paranoid group expressed the development of the belief in terms of worry. This is not entirely surprising if the content of the beliefs is considered. The beliefs of the paranoid group predominantly concern a 'negative self' concept or a paranoid idea, while those of the schizophrenics are largely 'positive self' or concern thought interference.

With respect to the reasons given for the development of the beliefs, one striking finding is that the majority of patients describe an abnormal 'internal state' as causally involved, including a majority of patients with paranoia or delusional disorder, who are thought not to be subject to abnormal experiences or to be very much less subject than their 'schizophrenic' counterparts. The criteria for delusional disorder (DSM III) specify that if hallucinations are present they should not be 'prominent'.

Interesting work is currently being conducted in gathering systematic accounts of 'prodromal' states, which identifies a sequence of psychological changes before clear psychotic symptoms such as delusions and hallucinations re-emerge (Birchwood 1992). In the patients interviewed here abnormal mood is uncommonly reported, while abnormal perceptual experiences are more frequent. However, while in the schizophrenic group these took the form of easily classified 'hallucinations', this was more difficult in the group with paranoia. Present-day models of hallucinations (for example Slade and Bentall 1988) emphasize the role of interpretation in a process previously regarded as more purely perceptual. This seemed consistent with some of the interview responses. It was noticeable, when discussing with subjects certain phenomena such as, for example, itching or pain, that it was difficult, if not impossible, to disentangle the sensory experience from the cognitive state of believing that some person or substance was responsible for the experience; there was no clear temporal sequence from the experience to the thought. The auditory experiences described by the schizophrenic subjects, in contrast, appeared to place a stronger emphasis on the sensory quality of the experience. However, these aspects were not systematically studied.

It is not clear why the apparently perceptual elements of experience should occur in different modalities, auditory in schizophrenics and olfactory and tactile in those with delusional disorder, although one important consideration is diagnostic: the nature of the experience described increases the probability of a particular diagnosis. Apart from this, are there other differences, such that the latter group seek explanations of abnormalities which are less bizarre than disembodied voices? (Smells and itching can both occur in the absence of a detectible source, while voices are perhaps less commonly present under such conditions.)

In Chapter 3 studies of reasoning in deluded and schizophrenic subjects were discussed. One processing style identified was the imposition of meaning on current experience employing strong prior expectations. Both at the stage of formation, and also in belief maintenance, the role of the 'external event' is perhaps relevant here. For the most part, the events described by the subjects were unremarkable (a GP changing a prescription, ambiguous comments made in the presence of the subject) and did not appear to lead necessarily from observation to belief.

Once the belief is formed, the vast majority of subjects report experiences or events which confirm them in their beliefs. Again the majority in both groups report internal states, mostly 'perceptual', although the paranoid subjects' responses are again somewhat harder to categorize as such, possibly indicating a stronger relative weighting of interpretation to sensory experience. External events are also reported, again events which generally do not seem compelling with regard to the truth of the hypothesis, and some of which may be regarded less as striking occurrences than as resulting from assiduous scanning of the environment for relevant material.

When asked whether they engage in seeking information, the members of the paranoid group are more likely to report this. That the nature of the information is confirmatory is not abnormal (see Chapter 2, the confirmation bias; for example Lord *et al.* 1979), although the information value of the data is perhaps abnormally poor. Few patients were prepared to consider that, even if the event cited had occurred (for example the patient's mother developing breathing difficulties), it was quite possible for the event to be true and yet the hypothesis false (that is for his mother, who was very elderly, to become ill and yet her GP not be trying to kill her). There is a clear failure of Bayesian reasoning in such instances; how abnormal such reasoning is (in terms of deviating from the actual performance of normals with strong beliefs), it is not possible to determine here, in the absence of an appropriate normal control.

There is some evidence that subjects who show an ability to reconsider the information value of their data as shown in response to hypothetical contradiction (Brett-Jones *et al.* 1987; Chadwick and Lowe 1990), are subsequently more likely to show improvement, whether spontaneously or in response to treatment. In this study only four subjects expressed a willingness to reduce conviction or reject their beliefs in response to a hypothetical contradiction, of whom two were among the three who had been willing to reconsider the informativeness of their data.

Most of the paranoid group and only one-third of the schizophrenic group reported acting on their beliefs. More recent work on the incidence of acting on delusions is reported by Wessely *et al.* (1993). It is not clear from this study what leads some patients to act in response to their beliefs and others not, nor why this should be more apparent (as was seeking evidence, another action) in the paranoid group. The data from the patients' psychiatrists indicate a trend towards the paranoids' beliefs being more stable and less treatable (by medication); perhaps these factors, or the more worrying quality of the beliefs, lead these patients to act on them. Buchanan *et al.* (1993), building on this work, have investigated further the relationship between delusional phenomenology and action in a mixed sample of psychotic patients. They found some interesting relationships: acting was associated with being aware of evidence for the belief and having sought out such evidence, with a reduction in conviction in response to hypothetical contradiction and, finally, with feeling worried (anxious, frightened, or sad) by the belief.

The differences between the two diagnostic groups should not be over-stated: they are modest. For many questions the groups showed no significant differences, and where differences occurred there was also a proportion of subjects from each group who fell into the same category. It is possible that the differences reflect not a dichotomy, but a dimension of severity of disruption of reasoning. This will be further discussed in Chapter 9.

The study cannot fully answer the question of whether the reasoning involved in the formation or maintenance (or both) of delusions is particularly abnormal. However, the nature of the data cited by subjects as causally responsible, both perceptual anomalies, in which reality discrimination is involved, and generally ambiguous events, suggests that at the formation stage subjects are forming strong beliefs too readily. Chapman and Chapman (1988) similarly found that some subjects reported experiences from which one would not reasonably infer their resultant beliefs. Employing confirmatory evidence to maintain beliefs is not itself abnormal; however, just as at the stage of formation, subjects in this study appeared to cite relatively weak evidence in support of their beliefs.

It did not prove possible to rate the bizarreness of subjects' belief statements reliably. Other researchers have also found this (Kendler *et al.* 1983; Flaum *et al.* 1991; Junginger *et al.* 1992), and the results add weight to the suggestion of Oltmanns (1988) that bizarreness is a problematic defining criterion of delusions and should be abandoned. (The DSM III-R criteria for schizophrenia include the presence of 'bizarre' delusions among other delusions.) Despite the problems with inter-rater reliability, it is perhaps of interest that each rater consistently rated the delusions of the schizophrenic group as more bizarre than those of the paranoid group, a finding also supported by Junginger *et al.* This may, however, simply reflect compliance with the diagnostic criteria. In terms of inherent implausibility, also regarded as characteristic of delusions (Mullen 1979), the inter-rater reliability was better but still not adequate ($x = 0.40$). Bizarreness and implausibility were very highly correlated, suggesting that the two dimensions are not conceptually distinct.

The belief content codings are predominantly 'positive self' and 'thought interference' for the schizophrenic group, and 'negative self' and 'paranoid' for the paranoid group (see p. 117). While, clearly, the nature of the delusion influences the diagnosis, it does not entirely determine it. For instance, the diagnosis of 'paranoia' allows for a wider range of delusions, and paranoid or negative self beliefs would not be ruled out by the diagnosis of schizophrenia. It is, however, possible that the sample was abnormal, especially in view of the substantial number drawn from a special hospital.

CONCLUSIONS

The findings of this study are consistent with the assertion of Chapman and Chapman that deluded subjects' reasoning about their delusions is not always reasonable:

The reasonableness of a belief should be judged in part by the range of evidence considered and by the weights given the various bits of evidence. The nondelusional person takes the usual step of considering more information about the world than the anomalous experience itself, while the delusional person responds to the experience as if it were the only datum available. (Chapman and Chapman 1988, 1976)

In the next chapter, a tentative new model of delusional belief formation will be outlined, which will draw on the existing literature together with the findings from the present study. In this model, a deficit of reasoning will be hypothesized to be one causal factor in delusion formation.

9 Towards a model of delusion formation*

INTRODUCTION

In this final chapter we summarize the principal findings of our work and present an outline of a new model of delusion formation which attempts to incorporate these findings. We illustrate the model with a case example. We also consider questions concerning the severity and chronicity of delusions and how our work relates to schizophrenia research.

CONCEPTS AND DEFINITIONS OF DELUSION

In Chapters 1, 4, and 5 the nature of delusions was considered. There has been a gradual shift, dating most notably from Strauss's (1969) paper, from viewing delusions as discrete entities, discontinuous with normal beliefs, to conceptualizing them as multidimensional phenomena which may be placed at various points along any given belief dimension, continuous with normality. The data presented in Chapters 4 and 5 supported this view, and we found that delusions are not always placed at the extreme point of a dimension, so that the usual defining characteristics are neither necessary nor sufficient, including even the most striking feature of delusions, high conviction. Oltmanns' (1988) description of delusions seems therefore to be the most accurate, if also the most open-ended.

The findings from the survey of the subjective characteristics of delusions (Chapter 5) identified subjective distress as a common feature of delusions, even in subjects without a primary affective disorder; this has not been previously much emphasized, and may have important theoretical and therapeutic implications. Conviction,

*This chapter incorporates revised versions of two previously published papers: Garety, P.A. (1991). Reasoning and delusions. *Br. J. Psychiat.*, **159**, (suppl. 14) 14–18 and Garety, P.A. (1992b). Making sense of delusions. *Psychiatry*, **55**, 282–91.

while undeniably characteristic, was not always absolute, and was shown, in Chapter 4, to fluctuate even in a subject whose delusions were regarded as 'fixed'. This suggests that delusions are not so unmodifiable (whether by experience or some other non-pharmacological factor) as previously thought, a hypothesis which is increasingly supported by cognitive behavioural intervention studies (for example Watts *et al.* 1973; Milton *et al.* 1978; Chadwick and Lowe 1990; Garety *et al.* in press).

The characteristic of delusions which is commonly taken to demonstrate clearly their irrational nature is incorrigibility. It was shown, in Chapter 2, that it is not always irrational to be incorrigible, and it is certainly not uncommon. Incorrigibility therefore represents another belief dimension, and its status as a defining characteristic of delusion, viewed in this light, is uncertain.

Two influential Jasperian views, the primary/secondary distinction and the irreducibility of primary or 'true' delusions, are subject to question (Winters and Neale 1983; Spitzer 1990). The frequency of primary delusions is unknown and the reliability of the distinction with secondary delusions poor. Its diagnostic significance is doubtful, and it is no longer being used in major standardized psychiatric assessment devices. The idea of the psychological irreducibility of true delusions has probably inhibited research this century into delusions (Matussek 1952). It appears likely that delusions are generally, if not always, secondary to some more basic dysfunction, given their occurrence in a wide variety of conditions. They frequently appear to be descriptions of, or explanations for, experience. The predominance of self-referent beliefs found in Chapter 5 is consistent with this view. Much recent work is proceeding on this assumption (for example Frith 1987; Oltmanns and Maher 1988). Spitzer (1990) has argued that when the experience in question is a person's own mental state, the resulting belief should not be called a delusion; this term should be reserved for statements uttered with subjective certainty and incorrigibility about the external world. However, while this is an interesting distinction, in practice it is not clear-cut. In the study described in Chapter 8 many subjects cited both internal mental states and external events as evidence for their beliefs; clearly, although plausible, these accounts may not be accurate descriptions of the actual process, and more work is needed here. From a theoretical perspective, cognitive biases, such as the probabilistic reasoning bias identified in Chapter 7, may give rise to abnormalities in the processing of both internal states of mind and external events: the association of both perceptual and reasoning biases in deluded subjects is consistent with this view.

Since delusions have until recently attracted relatively little interest as symptoms in their own right, methods of assessment have been limited. The application of the Personal Questionnaire method to delusions, described in Chapter 4, allows for more sensitive measurement of dimensions of interest, and has subsequently been used in longitudinal and intervention studies (Brett-Jones *et al.* 1987; Chadwick and Lowe 1990; Garety *et al.* in press).

Delusions have been categorized most frequently by content, and while this method yields a modest association with diagnosis this may be largely circular, since diagnostic systems specify common content areas. Some, influenced by Jaspers, have argued that content is irrelevant, in that it simply reflects the subject's pre-existing concerns, while others, often psychoanalysts, have argued, because this is so, that it is crucial. It is, however, not certain that pre-existing concerns are always expressed; rather some delusions seem to describe current experience. The formal structure of delusions has attracted some recent interest (for example Maher 1988) and attempts to classify by postulated cause have a long pedigree (see Chapter 1). Neither of these approaches has yet made much progress. An additional recurring interest has been the 'bizarreness' of a delusion. As we have noted, the reliability of assessments of bizarreness is generally poor, and proved again to be the case in the study reported in Chapter 8. It remains a possibility that bizarreness does reflect an important feature, but clearly reliability must first be improved.

Although comparisons between diagnostic groups were made in the studies presented here, no very striking differences between the groups were found. In the studies reported in Chapters 7 and 8, clear differences did not in general emerge. On none of the inference task variables were there significant differences between the schizophrenic and paranoid groups, and for most of the interview responses this was also true. Where differences were found, their theoretical implications are uncertain: they may not, for instance, reflect distinct disease entities or aetiologies, but, rather, different styles or stages of adaptation to a similar basic dysfunction. This will be discussed in more detail below.

TOWARDS A MODEL OF DELUSION FORMATION

In Chapter 6, theories of delusion formation were reviewed, and the experiment and interview studies in the subsequent chapters were designed to consider the role of a reasoning bias in delusion formation. In this section an attempt will be made to integrate the literature and evidence, and a tentative outline model of delusion formation will be presented. Since the focus of the work in this book has been the delusions of the non-affective 'functional' psychoses, the model will particularly address the formation of delusions in this category, although it is hoped that the model will also be capable of subsuming delusions associated with other diagnoses.

The review of the literature indicates that delusions are un-likely to share a common cause; their occurrence in such a wide variety of disorders provides strong support for this view. Where there is a clear neurological disturbance, for instance, causing clearly identifiable deficits and an apparently linked delusional belief, which disappears when the disturbance is treated, the cause appears evi-dent. However, even in such cases, if under the same conditions not all patients become delusional additional factors may need to be invoked. This requirement becomes increasingly pertinent as we move to considering the functional psychoses. Although the theory of delusions as accounts for anomalous perceptual experience is plausible, it is becoming clear that abnormal experience is not a sufficient condition, and may not even be necessary (Chapman and Chapman 1988).

The accumulating evidence for a judgemental bias in some deluded subjects also casts doubt on the determinant role of abnormal perception in all cases of delusion formation. Some deluded subjects are excessively influenced by current information, and make less use of past learned regularities in making inferences. They 'jump' to perceptions and to conclusions and express high conviction about their judgements.

The role of judgement has also been shown to be important in hallucinations, and it had been argued that hallucinations 'result from a dramatic failure of the skill of reality discrimination' (Slade and Bentall 1988, p. 214). It is proposed that hallucinators are more inclined than non-hallucinators to judge a perceived event as real and that they make rapid, over-confident judgements about their per-ceptions. In the study reported in Chapter 7, an association was found between rapid decision-making and the reported experience of perceptual anomalies. It was suggested that both delusions and hallucinations may arise from a common cause, a judgemental bias characterized by a failure to make use of past learned regularities.

However, an apparently contradictory bias has been reported in some deluded ('paranoid') subjects, a tendency to rely excessively on prior expectations when processing new information. One possibility is that there are two distinct groups, with different processing styles, which both result in delusions. In the reasoning experiment described in Chapter 7, with its 'neutral' content, strong prior expectations were not predicted. The role of such a processing style was not therefore examined in Condition 1 of the experiment. In Condition 2, which was designed to generate a belief held at high conviction, which would then be subjected to disconfirmation, it was possible to consider the role of prior expectations. However, neither the deluded subjects nor a sub-group of them appeared to be abnormally reluctant to change their hypotheses, perhaps because this relatively short task was not capable of generating an even 'normal' degree of incorrigibility, or because the excessively strong influence of prior expectations is more likely to occur with material which is not neutral.

An alternative possibility is that these two judgemental styles do not characterize two distinct groups of deluded subjects, but instead reflect two stages of response to an information-processing abnormality, or responses representing differing degrees of severity. In Chapter 6, Radley's (1974) proposal of a two-stage process was discussed. He suggested that 'paranoid' thinking results from a predisposition to employ 'cognitively simple' constructs, which are tightly organized but idiosyncratic. This may result in constructions which apply to only one facet of the situation, ignoring contradictory evidence. If, however, new evidence continually appears which cannot be integrated, the construct system may be progressively loosened, resulting in weaker predictions and thought disorder.

Arieti on the basis of his clinical observations makes a similar proposal:

The early paranoid who has delusions of persecution or of jealousy is able to foresee the future and direct his thoughts in logical chronological patterns that lead to the foreseen delusional deductions . . . . Later he becomes less logical, less capable of organising his thoughts in a logical series . . . his delusions become related to the *present time* [our emphasis] and not to the future, their content is not persecutory but more or less grandiose, and their emotional tone is shallower. Later his thinking presents definite scattering, his delusions are connected with the *immediate present* [our emphasis], and are of the definitely expansive type . . . . He accepts his delusions as indisputable, immediate reality, no longer caring to demonstrate logically their validity. (Arieti 1955, p. 245)

Hemsley (1990) also takes the view that subjects may change over time or that a severity dimension is represented, so that, given a biased reasoning style, at first it may be possible to maintain a stable delusional system in the face of limited disconformation, but that the system, encountering repeated failure, may be replaced by more transient belief systems characteristic of the non-paranoid schizo-phrenic. He quotes Anscombe (1987): 'less and less the subject forms his own impressions, and more and more he is impinged upon by his environment'.

An accumulation of 'non-fortuitous coincidences', as described by Arieti (1974) (cf. p. 79, Chapter 6) would, over time, make it less and less possible to integrate both normal and abnormal percepts within the subject's mental model of the world. The speed of this progression would be dependent on the severity of disturbance, and would correspond to Depue and Woodburn's (1975) observation of a change from 'paranoid' to 'non-paranoid' status with chronicity. This does not imply progression at the level of the presumed under-lying neural abnormality; for schizophrenia at least, the evidence is suggestive of a neurodevelopmental abnormality (cf. Murray *et al.* 1988). One implication of this is that therapy, both pharmacological and psychological, will be more effective if delivered early in the course of the disorder, before the individual has made numerous adjustments to both peripheral and core beliefs (cf. Quine 1953 in Chapter 2).

In Fig. 9.1 an attempt is made to integrate these ideas into a model of belief formation, highlighting those elements which are parti-cularly implicated in delusion formation. As we concluded in our review of theories of delusion formation and maintenance in Chapter 6, delusions are clearly complex phenomena, and it is likely that a number of factors contribute to their formation and maintenance. It is also probable that different types of delusions involve different mechanisms. The model we present here is therefore multifactorial and from it we would not attempt to derive group predictions. In some, personality, affect, self-esteem, and motivation play a part; in others, abnormalities of perception and judgement are prominent. Clearly, in some, a number of these different processes may operate as interacting causal mechanisms. Such a model, therefore, assists in making predictions only following a detailed assessment of the individual case, when abnormalities of particular processes have been identified.

Bentall (1990) has recently published an outline model of belief formation which bears some similarity to the model described here. Briefly, he proposes that beliefs generally arise from data in the world, which are perceived and about which inferences are made so that a belief is generated. Information search to corroborate or refute beliefs might then occur. Bentall proposes that delusions reflect abnormalities at one or more of these stages, although an abnormality at any par-ticular stage may be neither necessary nor sufficient for a delusion to

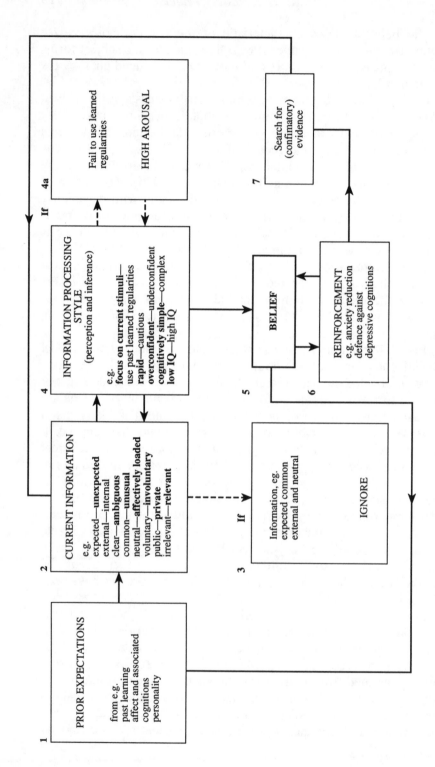

Fig. 9.1 A model of belief formation (with factors implicated in delusion formation in bold).

be formed. While similar, the model presented below is more detailed and emphasizes interacting processes to a greater extent.

In Box 1 (Fig. 9.1) the cognitive state of the person at the beginning of the process is represented. The subject starts with a set of prior expectations, derived from, for example, past learning, previous experiences, affective state, and accompanying cognitions, and personality traits. As has been emphasized in research in normal belief acquisition (for example Fischhoff and Beyth-Marom 1983; Alloy and Tabachnik 1984) prior expectations interact with new data in this process; data are not perceived 'cold'.

In this cognitive and affective state, the current information or datum (Box 2) is encountered. This information may vary along a number of dimensions: it may be more or less consistent with prior expectations; it may be internally or externally generated; it may be more or less clear; it may be common or unusual; it may be more or less affectively loaded; it may be relevant or irrelevant to current concerns; it may be experienced as voluntary/involuntary, or public/ private. The information may also concern two events, showing spatial or temporal contiguity. Much information we encounter is not extensively processed: if information is external, predicted, common, and affectively neutral, it may, after rapid preconscious processing, be ignored and processed no further (Dixon 1982) (Box 3). Other information will continue to be processed. In the interview study in Chapter 8 the majority of subjects reported both internal and external events as causative in their belief formation; their relative importance was not established.

The processing of the datum (perception and inference) (Box 4) will be influenced by the judgemental style of the individual (which may itself be influenced by the type of information being processed as discussed in Chapter 6). It is the judgemental style, and especially the extent to which subjects fail to make use of previously learned regularities, and focus excessively on prominent current stimuli, which is hypothesized to be particularly implicated in delusion formation in non-affective functional psychoses. Current situational information is accorded undue weight and inaccurate inferences result. It is also proposed that failure to make use of past learned regularities, which lead to expectancies, or 'response biases' (Hemsley 1990), frequently causes a mismatch between predicted and actual events and an increased state of arousal (Gray 1985). This state of high arousal (Box 4a) may then have further effects on judgemental style (such as rapid processing (Gray 1985)). Other relevant aspects of judgement include the extent to which subjects make rapid or cautious decisions (even if not in a state of high arousal), tend to over-/under-confidence in their judgements, attempt to integrate all information (are cognitively complex/simple), and intellectual ability. The relationship between these different aspects is at present not established, although Huq *et al.* (1988) found a positive correlation between rapid decision-making and over-confidence, and in the study reported in Chapter 7 an association was found between rapid decision-making and poorer verbal ability.

In this model, perception and inference have been presented as closely linked, and represented in the same box. Bentall separates them, but notes in his text that 'the clear distinction made between perception and inference . . . is in reality oversimplistic and perception is to some extent belief-driven' (Bentall 1990, p. 40). The role of inferential processes in perception has been noted frequently in this book, and similar aspects of judgemental style (for example rapidity or over-confidence) are relevant to both perceptual and other judgements.

The belief (Box 5) will result from the interaction of the information selected and the judgemental style. Where the information is very unusual and unambiguous, such as may be associated with a neurological deficit, so that no 'normal' explanation presents itself, a delusional belief may result, despite the application of 'normal' reasoning. (It may be, however, that repeated rather than one-trial exposure to the abnormal experience may be required for the normal arrival at an extraordinary explanation.) Maher's (1988) hypothesis of normal reasoning about abnormal experience may therefore apply, but in a more limited range of cases than he suggests. In conditions where the current information is, for example, ambiguous, the effect of a reasoning bias may be greater, so that the subject may form a hypothesis without taking reasonable account of past learning. As Chapman and Chapman comment: 'Delusional patients deny well established facts of physical reality that they and others have experienced all their lives.' (Chapman and Chapman 1988, p. 179). In this model model it is suggested that similar factors (reasoning style) might be responsible for both hallucinations and delusions.

It is also implied by the model, and by the literature reviewed in Chapter 2, that where current information is ambiguous and is relevant to pre-existing concerns, the individual's personality, affect, and motivation will exert a stronger influence on perception and judgement.

An early psychological account of perception by Blake and Ramsey makes a very similar point:

Briefly, the hypothesis is this: The stronger the hypothesis, the more will ambiguous information be suitable for confirming hypotheses. This implies, in short, that personality and motivational and experiential factors, having a maximum effect upon the kinds of hypotheses adopted, will therefore have a maximum effect upon the emergence of perception in situations where information is ambiguous. In other words, the personality of the individual enters more and more into the perception as ambiguity or his ignorance increases.

It is probable that a better way to state this is in the reverse, which is that the greater the ambiguity existing and the greater the ignorance, then the more it is necessary for the organism to create a strong hypothesis in order to maintain its equilibrium, its homeostasis, and to relieve it from anxiety concerning the potential threat which develops from its ignorance. (Blake and Ramsey 1951, p. 277)

If the information under consideration is puzzling, the arrival at a belief may be reinforced by its anxiety-reducing function, as Maher (1988) suggests (Box 6). Reinforcement may operate also under a number of other conditions, such as the arrival at a grandiose belief, defending a manic patient against depressive cognitions, as Neale (1988) has posited, or, similarly, a paranoid belief may protect a patient from depressive thinking (Zigler and Glick 1988).

The belief, which has now been formulated, will in turn influence the current state (Box 1) of the individual, modifying or reinforcing existing expectations (Alloy 1988), and potentially influencing the affective state and ultimately more enduring aspects of the personality, such as self-esteem.

Under certain circumstances, especially if the belief is novel, idiosyncratic, or unusual, there will then be a search for evidence (Box 7). This is normally (as discussed in Chapter 2 for normals, and as found in deluded subjects in Chapter 8) confirmatory in type. The prior expectations generated by the belief will now influence the selection of relevant current information (feedback from the belief, via Box 7 and via Box 1 to Box 2). The new information will be judged in the light of expectations, and predicted *relevant* data will be processed, rather than ignored. The belief will then be maintained by a process of repeated confirmation, and data are found which are to some extent plausibly confirmatory. A deluded person with a reasoning style which is rapid and over-confident, and who tends to ignore past learned regularities and conflicting information, may then maintain the belief with scant evidential support, as appeared to be the case for many subjects in the interview study (Chapter 8). Thus, the process of belief maintenance may be essentially 'normal' in seeking out confirmatory evidence and ignoring conflicting data, but with these processes exaggerated. As Chapman and Chapman propose, the delusional patients 'do not show a qualitatively unique kind of error, but instead accentuate a normal error tendency to the point of gross deviancy' (Chapman and Chapman 1988, p. 179). Here deluded subjects may therefore show an exaggerated 'top-downing', especially, in the earlier stages, or if less severely affected.

As we have discussed above (p. 128), this process of attempting to maintain a stable delusional system may break down over time, or may never be achieved with the more severe forms of disturbance. Thus, some individuals may have transient delusional beliefs, and, having met with repeated failure to incorporate evidence may no longer make predictions or attempt to structure their experience; bombarded with information, new beliefs are readily formed and equally readily discarded.

A CASE EXAMPLE

In order to illustrate the application of the model to an individual case, we present here a detailed assessment of a person with delusions, considering which different processes are implicated in the formation and maintenance of his delusions. This is also illustrated in Fig. 9.2.

The belief: the good and the bad aeroplanes
Brendan Bryan (a pseudonym) reported that aeroplanes were following him and, using their sophisticated instrumentation, were reading his mind and experimenting on him. He worried they might kill him. At times he felt suicidal about this, and had approached the police seeking legal action.

The development of the belief
Using the interview described in Chapter 8, the development of this belief was tracked. Mr Bryan related that the belief gradually formed in his mind at the time of his first 'breakdown' eight years before. At that time, his mood and thinking were both disrupted, in that he felt quite elated but also confused, and shortly after he started to notice planes that appeared to be following him. For some years, he thought he was simply under surveillance, but five years later, at the time of the breakdown of his marriage, when he had another relapse, he became convinced that the planes were directly interfering with his thoughts by putting thoughts into his mind. Over the years, he tested out these beliefs: he would go out to look for any planes that seemed to be following him. This activity resulted in daily confirmation of the belief: whenever he went out, planes could be seen in the sky, and sometimes they signalled to him, by turning suddenly.

Personal and psychiatric history
Mr Bryan, now aged 34, was born in India of Christian parents. He had a strict religious upbringing and attended a church school, where English was the language of study. His twin brother had a 'breakdown' at the age of 14

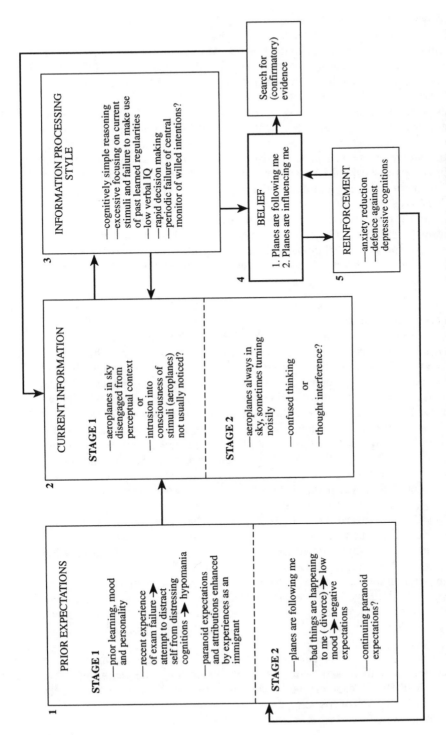

Fig. 9.2 A model of the factors involved in the formation and maintenance/change of BB's beliefs.

and was last known to be unemployed and wandering around France. His other brother lives near Brendan in London and works in an office.

Brendan was an average student at school and came alone to England at the age of 21 to train as an occupational therapist. He found the studies very difficult and eventually, after failing his exams and being admitted to hospital, was accepted to work at a lower level as a therapy aide. During this period he had an arranged marriage to a woman in India who was not informed of his psychiatric problems. His wife left him three years before our assessment, after four years of marriage. A year later, he was retired from work on medical grounds, having had approximately seven annual admissions to hospital. At the time of our assessment he had been out of hospital for one year and attended a psychiatric day centre.

Mr Bryan's first admission to a psychiatric hospital occurred while he was studying for his final exams, which he had already failed once before. He became overactive and sleepless and believed he had special powers from the Holy Spirit. He also thought planes were following him. He was elated. Subsequent admissions, however, were sometimes preceded by suicidal attempts and a depressed mood.

Current assessment

On inverview, Brendan reported that he was absolutely certain that the planes were following him, and that this was not a symptom of his illness, in the way that his past belief about the Holy Spirit was a symptom. He had been extremely preoccupied over the past week about the planes and very distressed; he felt 'terrified'. The evidence cited by Brendan for his belief was the daily presence of aeroplanes in the sky; he no longer felt compelled to look out for and note down the type of planes as he once had. He also said that some planes were bad, but others were 'good' and that he would miss these planes if they no longer followed him. Self-monitoring of conviction, preoccupation, and distress over the next week revealed that while conviction was maximal and unvarying, preoccupation and distress were greater when he was alone.

Mr Bryan's probabilistic reasoning was also assessed, following the procedure described in Chapter 7. His reasoning was clearly biased. In Condition 1, in which subjects are invited to ask for as much information as they need to reach a decision, Mr Bryan jumped to conclusions, making a decision on the basis of only *one* draw. In Condition 2, he appeared to be excessively influenced by the current stimulus: as each bead of a different colour was chosen, he changed his estimate to favour the jar with most beads of that colour, not making use of the information accumulating from the sequence of previous draws.

Finally, Mr Bryan's verbal intelligence was assessed. Despite having been educated in English, and, with difficulty studied for some years, his score on the Mill Hill Vocabulary Test was well below average, at about the tenth percentile for men of his age.

Formulation

Mr Bryan's belief that aeroplanes are influencing him developed over some years. It started at the time of his first psychotic episode and changed in content as he had further episodes. He appears to have experienced the symptoms of thought broadcasting and insertion at one stage. By then, Mr Bryan already believed that the planes were interested in him. What were the respective roles of prior expectation mood, abnormal experience, and reasoning in the formation of this belief?

The different factors postulated as involved in the construction of Mr Bryan's belief are represented in Fig. 9.2 drawing on the model of delusion formation given previously.

Mr Bryan's belief changed over time: the model considers the factors at Stage 1, when the first belief was formed, and at Stage 2, when it changed from the belief that he was being followed by the planes to believing that he was being influenced.

In Box 1, Stage 1, Mr Bryan's state before forming his belief is represented. As for any individual, he would start with a set of pre-existing expectations, mood states, and his unique personality. Recent experiences, such as being an immigrant and failing his examinations, would have further influenced his mood and expectations. It seems likely that in Mr Bryan's case, mood is very important. He had his first breakdown at the time of personal failure and first presented with symptoms of hypomania.

At the beginning, Mr Bryan's central delusion concerned having special powers from the Holy Spirit, and the belief about aeroplanes following him had an element of his being a special focus of attention. These may have served to distract him from the distress of exam failure, in the way that Neale (1988) proposes.

Cross-cultural factors may also be relevant. Westermeyer (1988) argues that both the structure and content of most delusions are not culture bound and that delusions can be readily identified across cultural boundaries. However, he notes that cultural change fosters paranoid delusions, in that, unsurprisingly, immigrants and refugees show high levels of paranoid ideation. It is therefore possible that Mr Bryan's recent experiences as an immigrant had engendered paranoid expectations and attributions. Recent research (Kaney and Bentall 1989) has also demonstrated that subjects with paranoid delusions show a characteristic attributional style, in which they make excessive external attributions for negative events.

The expectations influence the selection of information in the environment that is detected (Box 2). The principal evidence cited by Mr Bryan, at Stage 1, was the flying of aeroplanes overhead. It is not clear whether the perception of this was in any way abnormal. Were there perceptual changes at the time of his first episode, which caused the elements of the visual field to become separated from their context, so that aeroplanes, experienced as unexpected, became especially salient, in the way that Matussek (1952) proposed? Frith (1979) has also suggested that in schizophrenia percepts that

would normally be ignored arrive abnormally in consciousness and therefore demand an explanation. Possibly some such abnormality occurred when
Mr Bryan first noticed the aeroplanes.

In addition to the role of prior expectations, mood, and abnormal experience, there is evidence that Mr Bryan's reasoning showed characteristic
biases (Box 3). Mr Bryan offered no explanation of how the planes
influenced him: he seemed to require no account of the physical mechanism
that was operating, ignoring the ordinary physical realities that he otherwise
accepted. This is behaviour of the type that Chapman and Chapman (1988)
noted, in which the delusional person demonstrates a loss of the benefit of
accumulated life experience, accounting for a failure to reject delusional
beliefs as unrealistic. Here the reasoning is not entirely normal but, rather,
excessively cognitively simple (Radley 1974) and fails to make use of past
learned regularities. In addition to his uncritical acceptance of the extraordinary behaviour of the planes, there are also other indications of impov-
erished or biased reasoning. His assessed intellectual (verbal) functioning
was low, and his reasoning on the probabilistic task was biased toward a
rapid 'jump to conclusions' style and an over-emphasis on current stimuli.
This reasoning style would further facilitate the formation of hypotheses on
the basis of little information and would render more likely the ignoring of
past learning. Belief maintenance would also be affected by the biases.

The interacting combination of expectation (including mood), information, and the processing of that information, leads to Mr Bryan's belief: his
attempt to make sense of experience (Box 4). It is plausible, as Maher (1988)
suggests, that this arrival at an explanation, reducing anxiety-provoking
uncertainty, is reinforcing (Box 5). In this case also, the notion of being a
special focus of attention (at Stage 1) may have helped to bolster Mr Bryan's
flagging self-esteem in the face of failure, and might defend against
depression (Neale 1988). Mr Bryan reported that in the early stages he
sought confirmation of his belief: he looked out for aeroplanes. This
confirmatory activity is not itself abnormal: the confirmation bias is well
known in normals (Kahneman *et al.* 1982). However, in this case, where
a reasoning bias appeared to foster belief formation, it is also likely to
enhance belief maintenance on scant evidence.

However, the belief was not stable. We know that Mr Bryan's mood
deteriorated, the 'manic defence' possibly breaking down under the weight
of repeated negative experiences, including the major one of his divorce
(Box 1). In a depressed state, negative expectations of the world and the
future are common. Mr Bryan may also have continued to hold paranoid
expectations. In this state, at Stage 2, he encountered and selectively
attended to the environment (Box 2). He detected aeroplanes always in the
sky, often turning suddenly, apparently signalling to him. His thinking was
also experienced as subject to interference.

Frith (1987) proposes that symptoms of thought interference are a
consequence of a failure in the system whereby we monitor our intended
actions. If thoughts occur in the absence of this central monitoring, they
might be attributed to alien forces. This monitoring permits the distinction

between internally generated (willed) and externally generated (stimulus-elicited) actions.

How does this fit with Mr Bryan's symptoms of thought insertion and broadcasting? If the belief about aeroplanes following him had come after the report of the symptoms, the belief might be thought to explain them; however, these symptoms apparently occurred after the initial belief formation. They may in fact have partially resulted from the earlier delusional belief, rather than vice versa. Belief can drive perception and experience (Slade and Bentall 1988). Thus, when already believing that he was the special focus of attention of the aeroplanes and experiencing a further distressing life event (for example the end of his marriage), with a resultant lowering of mood and lack of clarity or 'confusion' in his thinking, Mr Bryan may have speculated on what role the planes were playing in this. Believing that the planes were doing bad things to him and feeling confused may in turn have led to an experience of interference with his thinking (rather than simply confusion) enhanced by a failure of the central monitor of willed intentions. In this way, prior expectations, abnormal experience, and a cognitive failure may have converged, resulting in the final, more stable belief that the planes are influencing his mind.

In this case example, therefore, we propose that Mr Bryan's delusional beliefs resulted from disturbances or deficits in a number of mechanisms: reasoning, affect, perception, and general cognitive functioning. We suspect that, in this case, perceptual biases are secondary to inference, but that affect is not secondary. We propose that information-processing disturbances combined and interacted with emotional distress to produce this man's delusions. Treatment along cognitive behavioural lines would therefore be most effective if both the affective and the cognitive mechanisms are addressed.

DELUSIONS AND SCHIZOPHRENIA RESEARCH

We have proposed here that one of the factors important to delusion formation is the 'reduced influence of past learned regularities'. This was derived from a model of the schizophrenia syndrome (Hemsley 1987), and was claimed to play a crucial role in a range of psychotic phenomena. Our present emphasis on the role of abnormal perceptions in the development of delusions made it inevitable that we should draw upon psychological models of schizophrenia. Such models frequently attempt to specify a single cognitive dysfunction, or pattern of dysfunction, from which the various abnormalities resulting in a diagnosis of schizophrenia might be derived. In contrast, the present model argues that a number of factors contribute to the formation of a single psychotic symptom, namely delusional belief. A similar approach may be taken for other phenomena such as hallucinations (cf. Slade and Bentall 1988). It is an empirical question whether a particular psychological abnormality contributes to more than one symptom. Our findings of an association between reasoning biases and perceptual disturbances (as in the study in Chapter 7) suggest that this is possible. A further difference of emphasis in the two approaches is that the present model proposes a dynamic interplay between the various factors. Models of schizophrenia tend to be more 'static' in their conceptualization of the disorder.

Psychological models of schizophrenia are currently attempting to link the proposed disturbances of information processing to their neural bases (cf. Gray *et al.* 1991*a,b*; Hemsley *et al.* 1993). It is therefore tempting to speculate on the possible biological bases of the phenomena for which we have been developing a model. We will resist the temptation; such an endeavour would be outside the scope of this volume. We note only the following: Squire (1992) proposes that 'In psychological terms the hippocampus contributes to the forming of new relationships such as those established when associating stimuli with their spatial and temporal context'. In similar vein, the neural network model of the functioning of the hippocampus and related brain structures developed by Schmajuk and his colleagues (for example Schmajuk and Tyberg 1990; Schmajuk and Thieme 1992) postulates a mechanism which prevents the formation of 'spurious associations'.

CONCLUDING REMARKS

In this little-researched area, almost everything remains to be done. The work presented in this book has necessarily been preliminary and exploratory, since psychological models of delusional thinking are at an early stage of development. More fruitful than wide-scale atheoretical data collection will be the refinement and testing of models of delusional thinking.

The role of affective states in delusional thinking has always been at the periphery of this book. However, the data have shown that even in subjects with non-affective psychoses, depression, or subjective distress may be prominent. Possible links between paranoid thinking, depression, and self-esteem are intriguing. The work of Bentall and Kaney and colleagues is stimulating much interesting research on the role of affect and attributions in delusions. To extend our work in reasoning biases, it would be interesting to compare deluded subjects with a primary depressive disorder with depressed non-deluded subjects and deluded non-depressed subjects on reasoning tasks. The content of the material employed should be varied, including neutral and affectively loaded tasks.

With respect to the development of the work described here, overcoming some of the limitations to the studies we have conducted is clearly desirable. The chief of these is to institute longitudinal studies of a variety of aspects of reasoning in people with delusions, in order to investigate the status of reasoning biases as causative. Given the multifactorial model we propose, cross-sectional group comparisons have clear limitations. Detailed single-case assessments as recommended by Shallice (1988) to detect biases/deficits in particular mechanisms using methods developed in neuropsychology, and to link this with detailed analyses of the delusion, may generate useful further hypotheses about the particular mechanisms likely to be disturbed for sub-types of delusions.

It is not clear to what extent a reasoning bias is present pre-morbidly. One possible approach to this question is to examine the reasoning style in the relatives of deluded subjects with an identified reasoning bias, for example assessing the extent to which relatives employ cognitively complex or simple constructs in making judgements.

The significance of the content of delusions remains unclear. In particular 'bizarreness', which is often regarded clinically as a characteristic feature, remains an unreliable concept. It is possible that if the concept were operationalized for reliable measurement it may have some interesting correlates. This is, however, at present entirely speculative.

We are intrigued by the possibility that causal perception is disrupted in some deluded subjects. If we accept White's (1990) suggestion that much of everyday causal processing is automatic, and makes use of the 'causal powers' of objects, then experimental tasks designed to measure this would be appropriate. Schlottman and Shanks (1992) have investigated the effects of varying contiguity and contingency on causal perception, employing a development of Michotte's (1963) classic 'launching' paradigm, involving collision between objects. Contiguity rather than 'past regularities' would be expected to exert a greater influence in some deluded subjects if the model outlined here is correct. In contrast with causal perception, causal attribution, as studied by Bentall, Kaney, and colleagues is, we suggest, a more complex process, operating at the 'controlled' rather than the automatic stage, and more open to influence by such factors as affect, personality, and other aspects of the environment.

Finally, the work we have described suggests that people with delusions are not 'irretrievably lost in untruth' as Jaspers so memorably averred; the formation rather than the maintenance of the delusion is thought to be more fundamentally disturbed. Developments in psychological therapy for delusions are encouraging (for example Garety *et al.* in press) and themselves generate new hypotheses about causal processes. The model we have proposed, while emphasizing the biases which lead to the formation of delusions, also has implications for the point at which interventions are delivered. Early intervention to help the person with delusions make sense of experience, and limit the progressive embedding of the delusion in a necessarily flawed mental model of the world, is indicated not only therapeutically but also on theoretical grounds.

In writing this monograph, we have noted in ourselves a tendency to selecting information consistent with our hypotheses and ignoring disconfirmatory evidence, which is similar to those processes we have suggested as relevant to delusions. We hope that in this case, this insight prevented the process becoming pathological and that the evidential support that we provide proves convincing to the reader.

Appendix 1 Reasoning about Delusions: A Structured Interview

R.A.D. STRUCTURED INTERVIEW

NAME ....

DATE OF INTERVIEW ....

INTERVIEWER ....

1. What is/are the belief(s)? (Not more than two)

A. .... `1–5, 7–9` [   ]

B. .... `1–5, 7–9` [   ]

2. Which of the two is more important, if two beliefs are given? `1–2,9` [   ]

3. How sure are you about X?
    Check: Do you have any doubts at all?

ABSOLUTELY	(100%) —
ALMOST CERTAIN	(90–99%) —
QUITE CERTAIN	(70–89%) —
HAVE SOME DOUBTS/NOT SURE	(40–69%) —
DOUBT IT	(less than 40%) —

    `5–1,8,9` [   ]

4. How do you feel about the possibility that X is not true?
    Is it at all possible? How likely is it?

ABSOLUTELY CERTAIN THAT X̄/	ABSOLUTELY IMPOSSIBLE THAT X̄	— (0%)
ALMOST CERTAIN	/VERY SMALL POSSIBILITY	— (1–10%)
QUITE CERTAIN	/POSSIBLE BUT IMPROBABLE	— (11–30%)
HAVE SOME DOUBTS	/SOME DOUBTS/50–50	— (31–60%)
DOUBT IT	/QUITE PROBABLE	— (more than 60%)

    `5–1,8,9` [   ]

5. How did all this start? What started you off thinking like this?

    Sudden realization —
    Gradual <u>worry</u> that X —
    Gradual entertaining of the possibility that X — `1–4, 7–9` [   ]
    Not possible to establish —

6. Did anything unusual happen to you? Did you see/hear/feel
    unusual things? How did you feel — happy, sad, etc.? (Note)

    Was an internal state involved YES/NO

1,2, 7–9	

7. What type of internal state? (Specify)

    Mood —
    Abnormal experience(s) —
    Other (specify) —
    None—

1–4, 7–9	

8. Did anything (else) unusual happen to you? Was anyone else
    involved? etc. (Note)

    Was an external event involved YES/NO

1,2, 7–9	

9. What type of external event? (Specify)

    Observable —
    Unobservable —
    Other (specify) —
    None —

1–4, 7–9	

10. You have told me how it started. Can you explain why you
    continue to think that X is so? Has anything happened since then?

    Any events/states since formation? YES/NO
    Any events/states in past week?

1–3, 7–9	

11. Return to Q.6.

    Has internal state been involved since formation? YES/NO

1,2, 7–9	

12. Return to Q.7.

    What type of internal state? (specify)

    Mood —
    Abnormal experience(s) —
    Other —
    None —

1–4, 7–9	

13. Return to Q.8.

    Have external events been involved since formation? YES/NO

1,2, 7–9	

14. Return to Q.9.

    What type of external event? (Specify)

    Observable —
    Unobservable —
    Other —
    None —

1–4, 7–9	

15. Do you at present (or have you in the past week) look for any evidence or information either to confirm/prove the correctness of your view or to test whether your view may be mistaken/disconfirm it?

    Any information search YES/NO

    | 1,2, 7–9 | |

16. What, if any, is the nature of the information or evidence? (Specify)

    Confirmatory —
    Disconfirmatory —
    Apparently irrelevant —
    None —
    Both confirmatory and disconfirmatory —

    | 1–5, 7–9 | |

17. In the light of this evidence/information, how likely is your view that X, how sure are you now that X?

    ABSOLUTELY CERTAIN   (100%) —
    ALMOST CERTAIN   (90–99%) —
    QUITE CERTAIN   (70–89%) —
    HAVE SOME DOUBTS/NOT SURE (40–69%) —
    DOUBT IT   (less than 40%) —
    NO EVIDENCE TO CONSIDER —

    | 5–1, 6–9 | |

18. Is it possible that this evidence/information could be true, and yet your belief not true? (Give example to explain). How likely is this?

    ABSOLUTELY CERTAIN THAT $\bar{X}$/ABSOLUTELY IMPOSSIBLE THAT $\bar{X}$ (0%) —
    ALMOST CERTIN   /VERY SMALL POSSIBILITY   (1–10%) —
    QUITE CERTAIN   /POSSIBLE BUT IMPROBABLE   (11–30%) —
    HAVE SOME DOUBTS   /SOME DOUBTS   (31–60%) —
    DOUBT IT   /QUITE PROBABLE   (more than 60%) —

    NO EVIDENCE TO CONSIDER —

    | 5–1, 6–9 | |

19. When you think about it now, is it at all possible that you are mistaken about X? YES/NO

    | 1,2, 7–9 | |

20. Is there anything/any evidence that might persuade you that you are mistaken? Let's see how we could test it.

    Let me suggest something hypothetical to you, which tests your view and you could tell me how you think you would react.

    Specify H.C. given _____

    _____

    Ignores or rejects relevance —
    Accommodates into system —
    Change level of conviction —
    Dismiss belief —
    Belief not testable, even hypothetically —

    | 1–5, 7–9 | |

21. Can you tell me about anything that you do, or do not do as a
     direct consequence of what you believe?

     Only code as yes if verified by staff/in case notes/by observation.
     YES/NO

1,2, 7–9	

Response sheet for subjects for questions 3 and 4

(a) How sure are you about your view?

          ABSOLUTELY CERTAIN   100% —
          ALMOST CERTAIN   90–99% —
          QUITE CERTAIN   70–89% —
          HAVE SOME DOUBTS/NOT SURE 40–69% —
          DOUBT IT   Less than 40% —

(b) How likely is it that your view is incorrect?

          ABSOLUTELY IMPOSSIBLE (THAT $\overline{X}$) 0% —
          VERY SMALL POSSIBILITY   1–10% —
          POSSIBLE BUT IMPROBABLE   11–30% —
          SOME DOUBTS/NOT SURE   31–60% —
          QUITE PROBABLE   More than 60% —

     or How sure are you that your view is incorrect?

          ABSOLUTELY CERTAIN (THAT $\overline{X}$) —
          ALMOST CERTAIN —
          QUITE CERTAIN —
          HAVE SOME DOUBTS —
          DOUBT IT —

Appendix 2 Notes on Reasoning about Delusions: A Structured Interview

Before starting see Case Notes and Staff. Elicit permission including permission to tape. Fill out demographic data sheet. Introduce self. Establish rapport, give explanation of purpose of interview ('to learn more about your current problems' etc.) and an indication of duration.

1. *Reach agreed statement of belief*
Probe for belief(s) with questions such as:

'I understand you've had something on your mind recently.'
'Has anything unusual been happening to you?'
'Dr X/Nurse X has told me that . . . .'

Show subject the statement(s) written down and ensure he/she agrees that it correctly represents his/her belief(s).

2. *Choose principal belief*
The one identified as most important by subject, or
the one most clearly listed in the case notes or by staff, or
the one most strongly held.

Try to agree principal belief which is to be rated throughout; if this is impossible continue with two beliefs (on two separate forms).
(Note if one or two beliefs to be coded.)

3. *Conviction/probability of X*
— 'how sure are you about X?'
probe: do you have no doubts at all?

Ask for a percentage estimate of certainty or ask to choose between listed categories (show form if preferred).

4. *Probability of $\overline{X}$*
Gently probe the subjects views about the possibility of the negation of his/her stated belief being true.
Ask for an estimate of its likelihood or ask to choose between listed categories (show form if preferred).

5–9. Belief acquisition

5. *Nature*
Assess the nature of the start of the belief — distinguish between a sudden realization in the form of a delusional perception or a more gradual onset. Distinguish between a growing *worry* and a growing *consideration* of the *possibility*. Note verbatim response.

6 and 7. *Internal state*
Was any kind of internal state involved in the initial formation of the belief? These must be reported by the subject as *cause* or appear to the interviewer as such.

— A mood state.
— An abnormal experience: auditory, visual, tactile, etc., hallucination, recognized by the subject as a *perceptual* experience regardless of his/her explanation for this.
— other.
Probe for subject's explanation of belief formation.

Note verbatim response and code later if preferred.

8 and 9. *External state/event*
Was any kind of external event involved, causally?
Was this event or evidence of the type which, in the correct circumstances, is capable of being verified by an individual other than the subject?
(even if it has not been).
Probe for subject's explanation of the belief formation.

10–14. Present maintaining factors

10. *Any factors?*
Is there anything, apart from the *initial* stated cause, which is at present maintaining the belief? Any more recent states or events?
Is there anything in the past week? (if so, Code 3)

11 and 12. *Internal state*
See 6 and 7

13 and 14. *External event*
See 8 and 9

15 and 16. *Information search*
Does the subject at present, or in the past week, look for any evidence to confirm or disconfirm his/her view. Assess whether there is any information search and, if so, its nature.

17 and 18. Information value of data

17. *Probability of belief given data*
If the subject offers any evidence ask him/her how likely the evidence renders the belief, using same five-point scale as Question 3 (show response sheet if preferred).

18. *Probability of $\overline{X}$ given data*
Ask also how likely it is that the belief may not be true even if that evidence is true. What is the probability of $\overline{X}$ — the belief not being true with this data being true? Use same five-point scale as Question 4 (show response sheet if preferred).

19. Possibility of being mistaken
Ask gently if the subject now considers it at all possible whether he/she is mistaken. Take simple yes or no response.

20. Response to hypothetical conviction
Discuss gently with subject how his/her belief might be tested. Suggest a hypothetical test, if at all possible, and ask how the subject *might* respond to such a test suggesting the falsity

of his/her view. Note verbatim response. Note if it proves impossible to think of a test of the belief and why.

21. Action
Ask the subject any actual behavioural change since belief formation in terms of comission or omission which is consequent on the belief. Only note yes if verified by staff/in case notes or by observation. (Do not include 'coming into hospital' — or changes in routine consequent on this unless this was volitional and as a direct result of the belief.)

Coding
The possible range of codes is given beside each question.
Codes 1–6 vary according to the possible responses given to each question.
Code 7 = response clear or understood but no coding available.
Code 8 = response ambiguous therefore don't know.
Code 9 = no response gained.

Appendix 3 List of Belief Statements

01 A woman talks to me without being present and sends me messages and photographs by special means, perhaps by telepathy
02 I am a royal personage and produce the money for the UK and the USA
03 I have a special mission to bring about world unity; I am the Lord two
04 My GP was trying to bait me through his ill-treatment of my mother
05 A BBC transmitter talks to me to drive me mad, and picks up my thoughts from my eardrums
06 People think I am a homosexual
07 The people in the ward are of a higher rank (in the army, RAF) than me; I'm the bottom of the pile
08 I am in danger of being killed because of what I know about the involvement of naval intelligence in an abortion racket
09 There is a secret organization responsible for the love, television, radio and newspapers; Charlie Kray controls it all
10 There is an offensive smell on the ward which is impregnating my clothes and hair so that I smell offensive
11 The Devil puts thoughts in my mind
12 People were following me around, saying bad things and planning to have intercourse with my wife
13 I think people know what I am thinking and can put thoughts into my mind
14 I am the illegitimate son of Albert Einstein
15 People in the street can tell about how I am feeling sexually
16 Ativan tablets damaged my heart and brain
17 I am pregnant; My mother is Queen Elizabeth I; I am the Son of God (Patient is male)
18 The CIA were setting me up and using me as a guinea pig
19 I have spiritual enlightenment only shared by Christ and the Buddha. I have been through the mystical circle
20 I have been under surveillance by the Vice Squad and the Inland Revenue
21 I am the Son of God
22 My feet smell offensive
23 There is a mind-reading computer in the village, driving me mad
24 I smell offensively of semen
25 I am the Messiah
26 A group of Rastas are planning to kill me (or beat me up)
27 I am part of a crime syndicate which is an organization in control of the world
28 I am suffering from syphilis in an advanced stage
29 I am the Son of God
30 I am infested with insects in my hair
31 The girl I am in love with causes 'planes to crash

References

Abroms, G.M., Taintor, Z.C., and Lhamon, W.T. (1966). Percept assimilation and paranoid severity. *Archives of General Psychiatry*, **14**, 491–6.

Alloy, L.B. (1988). Expectations and situational information as co-contributors to covariation assessment: a reply to Goddard and Allen. *Psychological Review*, **95**, 299–301.

Alloy, L.B. and Abramson, L.Y. (1979). Judgement of contingency in depressed students: Sadder but wiser? *Journal of Experimental Psychology: General*, **108**, 441–85.

Alloy, L.B. and Tabachnik, N. (1984). Assessment of covariation by humans and animals: the joint influence of prior expectations and current situational information. *Psychological Review*, **91**, 112–49.

American Psychiatric Association (1980). *Diagnostic and statistical manual of mental disorders* (3rd edn), (DSM III). APA, Washington.

American Psychiatric Association (1987). *Diagnostic and statistical manual of mental disorders* (3rd edn revised) (DSM III-R). APA, Washington.

Andreasen, N. (1984). *Scale for the assessment of positive symptoms* (SAPS). Department of Psychiatry, Iowa.

Anscombe, R. (1987). The disorder of consciousness in schizophrenia. *Schizophrenia Bulletin*, **11**, 241–60.

Arieti, S. (1955). *Interpretation of schizophrenia*. Robert Brunner, New York.

Arieti, S. (1974). *Interpretation of schizophrenia* (2nd edn). Crosby, Lockwood & Staples, London.

Arthur, A.Z. (1964). Theories and explanations of delusions: a review. *American Journal of Psychiatry*, **121**, 105–15.

Asberg, M., Montgomery, S., Perris, C., Schalling, D., and Sedvall, G. (1978). The comprehensive psychopathological rating scale. *Acta Psychiatrica Scandinavica*, Suppl. 271, 5–27.

Bannister, D. (1960). Conceptual structure in thought-disordered schizophrenics. *Journal of Mental Science*, **108**, 825–42.

Barber, T.X. and Calverley, D.S. (1964). An experimental study of 'hypnotic' (auditory and visual) hallucinations. *Journal of Abnormal and Social Psychology*, **63**, 13–20.

Baruch, I., Hemsley, D.R., and Gray, J.A. (1988). Differential performance of acute and chronic schizophrenics in a latent inhibition task. *Journal of Nervous and Mental Disease*, **176**, 598–606.

Benson, D.F. and Stuss, D.T. (1990). Frontal Lobe influences on delusions: a clinical perspective. *Schizophrenia Bulletin*, **16**, 403–11.

Bentall, R.P. (1990). The syndromes and symptoms of psychosis Or why you can't play 'twenty questions' with the concept of schizophrenia and hope to win. In *Reconstructing schizophrenia* (ed. R.P. Bentall) pp. 23–60, ch. 2. Routledge, London.

Bentall, R.P., Jackson, H.F., and Pilgrim, D. (1988). Abandoning the concept of 'schizophrenia': some implications of validity arguments for psychological research into psychotic phenomena. *British Journal of Clinical Psychology*, **27**, 303–24.

Bentall, R.P., Kaney, S., and Dewey, M.E. (1991). Paranoia and social reasoning: an attribution theory analysis. *British Journal of Clinical Psychology*, **30**, 13–23.

Berkowitz, R. (1981). The distinction between paranoid and non-paranoid forms of schizophrenia. *British Journal of Clinical Psychology*, **20**, 15–23.

Berner, P., Gabriel, E., and Schanda, H. (1980). Non-schizophrenic paranoid syndromes. *Schizophrenia Bulletin*, **6**, 627–32.

Berrios, G. (1991). Delusions as 'wrong beliefs': a conceptual history. *British Journal of Psychiatry*, **159**, (Suppl. 14), 6–13.

Birchwood, M. (1992). Early intervention in schizophrenia: Theoretical background and clinical strategies. *British Journal of Clinical Psychology*, **31**, 257–78.

Blake, R.R. and Ramsey, G.V. (1951). *Perception — an approach to personality*. Ronald Press, New York.

Bleuler, E. (1906). *Affectivität, Suggestibilität, Paranoia*. Halle, Marhold.

Bleuler, E. (1911). *Dementia praecox or the group of schizophrenias* (trans. I. Zinkin, 1950). International University Press, New York.

BMDP (1988). *BMDP statistical software manual*. BMDP, Los Angeles.

Boyle, M. (1990). *Schizophrenia — a scientific delusion?* Routledge, London.

Brennan, J.H. and Hemsley, D.R. (1984). Illusory correlations in paranoid and non-paranoid schizophrenia. *British Journal of Clinical Psychology*, **23**, 225–6.

Brett-Jones, J., Garety, P.A., and Hemsley, D. (1987). Measuring delusional experiences: a method and its application. *British Journal of Clinical Psychology*, **26**, 257–65.

Brockington, I.F., Kendell, R.E., Wainwright, R.S., Hillier, V.F., and Walker, J. (1979). The distinction between the affective psychoses and schizophrenia. *British Journal of Psychiatry*, **135**, 243–8.

Broga, M.I. and Neufeld, R.W. (1981). Multivariate cognitive performance levels and response styles among paranoid and non-paranoid schizophrenics. *Journal of Abnormal Psychology*, **90**, 495–509.

Buchanan, A., Reed, A., Wessely, S., Garety, P., Taylor, P., Grubin, D., and Dunn, G. (1993). Acting on delusions (2): the phenomenological correlates of acting on delusions. *British Journal of Psychiatry*, **163**, 77–81.

Butler, R.W. and Braff (1991). Delusions: a review and integration. *Schizophrenia Bulletin*, **17**, 633–47.

Cameron, N. (1951). Perceptual organisation and behaviour pathology. In *Perception: an approach to personality* (ed. R.R. Blake and G.V. Ramsey) pp. 283–306. Ronald Press, New York.

Chadwick, P. and Lowe, C. (1990). The measurement and modification of delusional beliefs. *Journal of Consulting and Clinical Psychology*, **58**, 225–32.

Chapman, L.J. (1967). Illusory correlations in observational report. *Journal of Verbal Learning and Verbal Behaviour*, **6**, 151–5.

Chapman, L.J. and Chapman, J.P. (1959). Atmosphere effect re-examined. *Journal of Experimental Psychology*, **58**, 220–6.

Chapman, L.J. and Chapman, J.P. (1973). *Disordered thought in schizophrenia*. Appleton-Century-Crofts, New York.

Chapman, L.J. and Chapman, J.P. (1980). Scales for rating psychotic and psychotic like experiences as continua. *Schizophrenia Bulletin*, **6**, 476–89.

Chapman, L.J. and Chapman, J.P. (1988). The genesis of delusions. In *Delusional beliefs* (ed. T.F. Oltmanns and B.A. Maher) pp. 167–83, ch. 8. Wiley, New York.

Chapman, L.J., Chapman, J.P., and Raulin, M.L. (1978). Body-image aberration in schizophrenia. *Journal of Abnormal Psychology*, **87**, 399–407.

Christodoulou, G.N. (1986). Course and outcome of delusional misidentification syndromes. *Bibliotheca Psychiatrica*, **164**, 143–8.

Clark, D.A. (1984). Psychophysiological, behavioural and self-report investigation into the cognitive-affective interaction within the context of potentially aversive ideation. Unpublished PhD. Institute of Psychiatry, University of London.

Cohen, J. (1960). A coefficient of agreement for nominal scales. *Educational and Psychological Measurement*, **20**, 37–46.

Cohen, J. (1968). Weighted kappa: nominal scale agreement with provision for scaled disagreement or partial credit. *Psychological Bulletin*, **70**, 213–20.

Colbourn, L.J. and Lishman, W.A. (1979). Lateralisation of functions and psychotic illness: a left hemisphere deficit? In *Hemisphere asymmetries of function in psychopathology* (ed. J. Gruzelier and P. Flor-Henry) pp. 539–60. Elsevier, Amsterdam.

Cooper, A.F., Kay, D.W.K., Curry, A.R., Garside, R.F., and Roth, M. (1974). Hearing loss in paranoid and affective disorders of the elderly. *Lancet*, **2**, 851–4.

Cummings, J.L. (1985). Organic delusions. *British Journal of Psychiatry*, **146**,. 184–97.

Cutting, J. (1985). *The psychology of schizophrenia*. Churchill Livingstone, Edinburgh.

Cutting, J. (1987). The phenomenology of acute organic psychosis. Comparison with acute schizophrenia. *British Journal of Psychiatry*, **151**, 324–32.

Cutting, J. (1991). Delusional misidentification and the role of the right hemisphere in the appreciation of identity. *British Journal of Psychiatry*, **159**, (Suppl. 14), 70−5.

David, A.S. (1987). Tachistoscopic tests of colour naming and matching in schizophrenia: evidence of posterior collosum dysfunction? *Psychological Medicine*, **17**, 621−30.

Depue, R.A. and Woodburn, L. (1975). Disappearance of paranoid symptoms with chronicity. *Journal of Abnormal Psychology*, **84**, 84−6.

Dickstein, L.S. (1978). Error processes in syllogistic reasoning. *Memory and Cognition*, **6**, 537−43.

Dixon, N.F. (1982). *Preconscious processing*. Wiley, Chichester.

Dupré, E. and Logre, J. (1911). Confabulatory delusional states (Les délires d'imagination). *Encéphale*, **6a**, 209−32 (In *The clinical roots of the schizophrenia concept*, 1987, (trans. J. Cutting and M. Shepherd) Cambridge University Press.)

Eckblad, M. and Chapman, L.J. (1983). Magical ideation as an indicator of schizoptypy. *Journal of Consulting and Clinical Psychology*, **51**, 215−25.

Edwards, W. (1954). The theory of decision making. *Psychological Bulletin*, **51**, 380−417.

Edwards, W. (1982). Conservatism in human information processing. In *Judgement under uncertainty: heuristics and biases* (ed. D. Kahneman, P. Slovic, and A. Tversky) pp. 359−69. Cambridge University Press.

Einhorn, H.J. and Hogarth, R.M. (1978). Confidence in judgment: persistence of the illusion of validity. *Psychological Review*, **85**, 395−416.

Einhorn, H.J. and Hogarth, R.M. (1981). Behavioural decision theory: processes of judgment and choice. *Annual Review of Psychology*, **32**, 53−88.

Einhorn, H.J. and Hogarth, R.M. (1986). Judging probable cause. *Psychological Bulletin*, **99**, 3−19.

Ellis, H.D. and Young, A.W. (1990). Accounting for delusional misidentifications. *British Journal of Psychiatry*, **157**, 239−48.

Erickson, J.R. (1974). A set analysis of behaviour in formal syllogistic reasoning tasks. In *Theories in cognitive psychology: the Loyola Symposium* (ed. R. Solso) pp. 305−29. Erlbaum, Hillsdale, NJ.

Estes, W.K. (1976). The cognitive side of probability learning. *Psychological Review*, **83**, 37−64.

Evans, J. St B.T. (1980). Current issues in the psychology of reasoning. *British Journal of Psychology*, **71**, 227−39.

Evans, J. St B.T. (1982). *The psychology of deductive reasoning*. Routledge & Kegan Paul, London.

Everitt, B.S. (1980). *Cluster analysis* (2nd edn). Garner, London.

Feighner, J.P., Robins, E., and Guze, S.B. (1972). Diagnostic criteria for use in psychiatric research. *Archives of General Psychiatry*, **26**, 57−63.

Fischhoff, B. and Beyth-Marom, R. (1983). Hypothesis evaluation from a Bayesian perspective. *Psychological Review*, **90**, 239−60.

Fischhoff, B., Slovic, P., and Lichtenstein, S. (1977). Knowing with certainty: the appropriateness of extreme confidence. *Journal of Experimental Psychology: Human Perception and Performance*, **3**, 552–64.

Flaum, M., Arndt, S., and Andreasen, N.C. (1991). The reliability of 'bizarre' delusions. *Comprehensive Psychiatry*, **32**, 59–65.

Fleiss, J.L. (1986). *The design and analysis of clinical experiments*. Wiley, New York.

Folstein, M. and Luria, R. (1973). Reliability, validity and clinical application of the visual analogue mood scale. *Psychological Medicine*, **3**, 479–86.

Forgus, R.H. and De Wolfe, A.S. (1974). Coding of cognitive input in delusional patients. *Journal of Abnormal Psychology*, **83**, 278–84.

Foulds, G.A. and Bedford, A. (1975). Hierarchy of classes of personal illness. *Psychological Medicine*, **5**, 181–92.

Freedman, A., Kaplan, H., and Sadock, B. (1975). *Comprehensive textbook of psychiatry* (2nd edn). Williams & Wilkins, Baltimore.

Freeman, T. (1981). On the psychopathology of persecutory delusions. *British Journal of Psychiatry*, **139**, 529–32.

Freeman, T. (1990). Psychoanalytic aspects of morbid jealousy in women. *British Journal of Psychiatry*, **156**, 68–72.

French, C.C. (1992). Factors underlying belief in the paranormal: do sheep and goats think differently? *The Psychologist*, **5**, 295–9.

Freud, S. (1915). A case of paranoia running counter to the psychoanalytic theory of the disease. In *Collected papers*, Vol. 2, (1956). Hogarth Press, London.

Frith, C.D. (1979). Consciousness, information processing and schizophrenia. *British Journal of Psychiatry*, **134**, 225–35.

Frith, C.D. (1987). The positive and negative symptoms of schizophrenia reflect impairments in the perception and initiation of action. *Psychological Medicine*, **17**, 631–48.

Frith, C.D. and Done, D.J. (1989). Experiences of alien control in schizophrenia reflect a disorder in the central monitoring of action. *Psychological Medicine*, **19**, 359–63.

Fulford, K.W.M. (1989). *Moral theory and medical practice*. Cambridge University Press.

Gallup, G.H. and Newport, F. (1991). Belief in paranormal phenomena among adult Americans. *Skeptical Inquirer*, **15**, 137–46.

Garety, P.A. (1985). Delusions: problems in definition and measurement. *British Journal of Medical Psychology*, **58**, 25–34.

Garety, P.A. (1990). Reasoning rationality and delusion: studies in the concepts, characteristics and rationality of delusions. Unpublished PhD thesis. University of London.

Garety, P. (1991). Reasoning and delusions. *British Journal of Psychiatry*, **159** (Suppl. 14), 14–18.

Garety, P.A. (1992*a*). Assessment of symptoms and behaviour. In *Innovations in the psychological management of schizophrenia* (ed. M. Birchwood and N. Tarrier) pp. 3–20, ch. 1. Wiley, Chichester.

Garety, P.A. (1992*b*). Making sense of delusions. *Psychiatry*, **55**, 282–91.

Garety, P.A. and Hemsley, D.R. (1987). Characteristics of delusional experience. *European Archives of Psychiatry and Neurological Sciences*, **236**, 294–8.

Garety, P.A. and Wessely, S. (1994). The assessment of positive symptoms. In *Assessment procedures for the psychoses* (ed. T.R.E. Barnes and H. Nelson) pp. 21–39, ch. 3. Chapman and Hall, London.

Garety, P.A., Everitt, B.S., and Hemsley, D.R. (1988). The characteristics of delusions: a cluster analysis of deluded subjects. *European Archives of Psychiatry and Neurological Sciences*, **237**, 112–14.

Garety, P.A., Hemsley, D.R., and Wessely, S. (1991). Reasoning in deluded schizophrenic and paranoid patients: biases in performance on a probabilistic inference task. *Journal of Nervous and Mental Disease*, **179**, 194–201.

Garety, P.A., Kuipers, L., Fowler, D., Chamberlain, F., and Dunn, G. Cognitive behavioural therapy for drug resistant psychosis. *British Journal of Medical Psychology*. (In press.)

Gholson, B. and Barker, P. (1985). Kuhn, Lakatos and Laudan. Applications in the history of physics and psychology. *American Psychologist*, **40**, 755–69.

Gray, J.A. (1985). A whole and its parts: behaviour, the brain, cognition and emotion. *Bulletin of the British Psychological Society*, **38**, 99–112.

Gray, J.A., Feldon, J., Rawlins, J.N.P., Hemsley, D.R., and Smith, A.D. (1991*a*). The neuropsychology of schizophrenia. *Behavioral and Brain Sciences*, **14**, 1–84.

Gray, J.A., Hemsley, D.R., Gray, N., Feldon, J., and Rawlins, J.N.P. (1991*b*). Schizophrenia bits: misses, mysteries and hits. *Behavioral and Brain Sciences*, **14**, 56–84.

Grossman, A. (1989). Single-case longitudinal studies investigating the relationship between delusional beliefs and mood state. Unpublished MSc thesis. Institute of Psychiatry, University of London.

Gruhle, H.W. (1915). Selbstschilderung und Einfuhlung. *Zeitschrift fur die Gesamte Neurologie und Psychiatrie*, **28**, 148–231.

Gudeman, H.E. (1966). The phenomenology of delusions. *Review of Existential Psychology & Psychiatry*, **6**, 196–210.

Hall, J.N. (1974). Inter-rater reliability of ward rating scales. *British Journal of Psychiatry*, **125**, 248–55.

Harper, D.J. (1992). Defining delusions and the serving of professional interests: the case of 'paranoia'. *British Journal of Medical Psychology*, **65**, 357–70.

Harre, R. and Madden, E.H. (1975). *Causal powers: a theory of natural necessity*. Blackwell, Oxford.

Harrow, M., Rattenbury, F., and Stoll, F. (1988). Schizophrenic delusions: an analysis of their persistence, of related premorbid ideas, and of three major dimensions. In *Delusional beliefs* (ed. T.E. Oltmanns and B.A. Maher) pp. 184–211. Wiley, New York.

Hartman, L.M. and Cashman, F.E. (1983). Cognitive behavioural and psychopharmacological treatment of delusional symptoms: a preliminary report. *Behavioural Psychotherapy*, **11**, 50–61.

Heilbrun, A.B. (1975). A proposed basis for delusion formation within an information processing model of paranoid development. *British Journal of Social and Clinical Psychology*, **14**, 63–71.

Heilbrun, A.B. and Bronson, N. (1975). The fabrication of delusional thinking in normals. *Journal of Abnormal Psychology*, **84**, 422–5.

Heilbrun, A.B. and Heilbrun, K.S. (1977). Content analysis of delusions in reactive and process schizophrenics. *Journal of Abnormal Psychology*, **86**, 597–608.

Hemsley, D.R. (1982). Cognitive impairment in schizophrenia. In *The pathology and psychology of cognition* (ed. A. Burton) pp. 169–203. Methuen, London.

Hemsley, D.R. (1987). An experimental psychological model for schizophrenia. In *Search for the causes of schizophrenia* (ed. H. Hafner, W.F. Gattaz, and W. Janzarik) pp.179–88. Springer, Heidelberg.

Hemsley, D.R. (1988). Information processing and schizophrenia. In *Schizophrenia: concepts, vulnerability, and intervention* (ed. E. Straube and K. Hahlweg) pp. 59–76. Springer, Heidelberg.

Hemsley, D.R. (1990). What have cognitive deficits to do with schizophrenia? In *Weissenauer schizophrenia symposium No. 8* (ed. G. Huber) pp. 111–27. Schattauer, Stuttgart.

Hemsley, D.R. and Garety, P.A. (1986). Formation and maintenance of delusions: a Bayesian analysis. *British Journal of Psychiatry*, **149**, 51–6.

Hemsley, D.R., Rawlins, J.N.P., Feldon, J., Jones, S.H., and Gray, J.A. (1993). The neuropsychology of schizophrenia: act 3. *Behavioural and Brain Sciences*, **16**, 209–15.

Hoenig, J. (1968). The clinical usefulness of the phenomenology of delusion. *International Journal of Psychiatry*, **6**, 41–5.

Hole, R.W., Rush, A.J., and Beck, A.T. (1979). A cognitive investigation of schizophrenic delusions. *Psychiatry*, **42**, 312–19.

Hollon, S.D. and Bemis, K.M. (1981). Self-report and the assessment of cognitive functions. In *Behavioral assessment*. (ed. M. Hersen and A.S. Bellack) pp. 125–74. Pergamon, New York.

Horowitz, J.M. (1978). *Image formation and cognition* (2nd edn). Appleton-Century-Crofts, New York.

Hume, D. (1739/1964). *A treatise of human nature*. Scientia, Aalen.

Huq, S.F., Garety, P.A., and Hemsley, D.R. (1988). Probabilistic judgements in deluded and non-deluded subjects. *Quarterly Journal of Experimental Psychology*, **40A**, 801–12.

Jaspers, K. (1913). *General psychopathology* (trans. J. Hoenig and M.W. Hamilton, 1959). Manchester University Press.

Johnson, M.K. (1988). Discriminating the origin of information. In *Delusional beliefs* (ed. T.F. Oltmanns and B.A. Maher) pp. 34–65. Wiley, New York.

Johnson, M.K. and Raye, C.L. (1981). Reality monitoring. *Psychological Review*, **88**, 67–85.

Johnson, M.K., Raye, C.L., Foley, H.J., and Foley, M.A. (1981). Cognitive operations and decision bias in reality monitoring. *American Journal of Psychology*, **91**, 37–64.

Johnson, W.G., Ross, J.M., and Mastria, M.A. (1977). Delusional behaviour: an attributional analysis of development and modification. *Journal of Abnormal Psychology*, **86**, 421–6.

Johnson-Abercrombie, M.L. (1960). *The anatomy of judgement*. Basic Books, New York.

Johnson-Laird, P.N. (1982). Thinking as a skill. *Quarterly Journal of Experimental Psychology*, **34A**, 1–29.

Johnson-Laird, P.N. (1983). *Mental models: towards a cognitive science of language, inference and consciousness*. Cambridge University Press.

Johnson-Laird, P.N. and Bara, B.G. (1984). Syllogistic inference. *Cognition*, **16**, 1–61.

Jolliffe, I.T. (1986). *Principal component analysis*. Springer, New York.

Jones, E.E., Kanouse, D.E., Kelley, H.E., Nisbett, R.E., Valins, S., and Weiner, B. (ed.) (1972). *Attributions: perceiving the causes of behaviour*. General Learning Press, Morristown, NJ.

Jones, S.H., Hemsley, D.R., and Gray, J.A. (1992). Loss of the Kamin blocking effect in acute but not chronic schizophrenics. *Biological Psychiatry*, **32**, 739–55.

Junginger, J., Barker, S., and Coe, D. (1992). Mood theme and bizarreness of delusions in schizophrenia and mood psychosis. *Journal of Abnormal Psychology*, **101**, 287–92.

Kahneman, D. and Tversky, A. (1973). On the psychology of prediction. *Psychological Review*, **80**, 251–73.

Kahneman, D., Slovic, P., and Tversky, A. (ed.) (1982). *Judgement under uncertainty: heuristics and biases*. Cambridge University Press, New York.

Kamin, L.J. (1969). Predictability, surprise, attention and conditioning. In *Punishment and aversive behaviour* (ed. B.A. Campbell and R.M. Church) pp. 279–96. Appleton-Century-Crofts, New York.

Kaney, S. and Bentall, R. (1989). Persecutory delusions and attributional style. *British Journal of Medical Psychology*, **62**, 191–8.

Kay, D.W.K., Cooper, A.F., Garside, R.F., and Roth, M. (1976). The differentiation of paranoid from affective psychoses by patients' premorbid characteristics. *British Journal of Psychiatry*, **129**, 207–15.

Kay, S., Fiszbein, A., and Opler, L. (1987). The positive and negative syndrome scale for schizophrenia (PANSS). *Schizophrenia Bulletin*, **13**, 261–75.

Kelley, H.H. (1967). Attribution theory in social psychology. In *Nebraska symposium on motivation* (ed. D. Levine) pp. 192–240. University of Nebraska Press, Lincoln.

Kelley, H.H. (1973). The process of causal attribution. *American Psychologist*, **28**, 107–28.

Kelly, G.A. (1955). *A theory of personality: the psychology of personal constructs*. Norton, New York.

Kendell, R.E. and Brockington, I.F. (1980). The identification of disease entities and the relationship between schizophrenic and affective psychoses. *British Journal of Psychiatry*, **137**, 324–31.

Kendler, K. (1984). Paranoia (delusional disorder). *Trends in Neuroscience*, **7**, 14–17.

Kendler, K.S., Glazer, W.M., and Morgenstern, H. (1983). Dimensions of delusional experience. *American Journal of Psychiatry*, **140**, 466–9.

Kihlstrom, J.F. and Hoyt, I.P. (1988). Hypnosis and the psychology of delusions. In *Delusional beliefs* (ed. T.F. Oltmanns and B.A. Maher) pp. 66–109. Wiley, New York.

Knight, R.A. (1984). Converging models of cognitive deficit in schizophrenia. In *Theories of schizophrenia and psychosis. Nebraska Symposium on motivation, 1983* (ed. W.D. Spaulding and J.K. Cole) pp. 93–156. University of Nebraska Press, Lincoln.

Kraepelin, E. (1899). Dementia praecox and paraphrenia. In *Textbook of psychiatry* (8th German edn), (trans. R.M. Bradley, ed. G.M. Robertson, 1919), Vol. III, Pt. II. Livingstone, Edinburgh.

Kraweicka, M., Goldberg, D., and Vaughan, M. (1977). A standardised psychiatric assessment scale for rating chronic psychotic patients. *Acta Psychiatrica Scandinavica*, **55**, 299–308.

Kretschmek, E. (1927). *Der sensitive Beziehungswahn*. Springer, Berlin.

Kuhn, T.S. (1962). *The structure of scientific revolutions*. University of Chicago Press.

Kulick, A.R., Harrison, G.P., and Keck, P.E. (1990). Lycantropy and self-identification. *Journal of Nervous and Mental Disease*, **178**, 134–7.

Lacan, J. (1932). The case of Aimée, or self-punitive paranoia. In *The clinical roots of the schizophrenia concept* (trans. J. Cutting and M. Shepherd (ed.) pp. 213–27, 1987). Cambridge University Press.

Lakatos, I. (1970). Falsification and the methodology of scientific research programmes. In *Criticism and the growth of knowledge* (ed. I. Lakatos and A. Musgrave) pp. 91–198. Cambridge University Press.

Levy, R. and Maxwell, A.E. (1968). The effect of verbal context on the recall of schizophrenics and other psychiatric patients. *British Journal of Psychiatry*, **114**, 311–16.

Lichtenstein, S. and Fischhoff, B. (1977). Do those who know more also know more about how much they know? The calibration of probability judgements. *Organisational Behaviour and Human Performance*, **20**, 159–83.

Lichtenstein, S., Fischhoff, B., and Phillips, L.D. (1982). Calibration of probabilities: the state of the art to 1980. In *Judgement under uncertainty: heuristics and biases* (ed. D. Kahneman, P. Slovic, and A. Tversky) pp. 306–34. Cambridge University Press, New York.

Liddle, P.F. and Morris, D.L. (1991). Schizophrenic syndromes and frontal lobe performance. *British Journal of Psychiatry*, **158**, 340–5.

Lord, C., Lepper, M.R., and Ross, L. (1979). Biased assimilation and attitude polarisation: the effects of prior theories on subsequently considered evidence. *Journal of Personality and Social Psychology*, **37**, 2098–110.

Lubow, R.E., Weiner, I., and Feldon, J. (1982). An animal model of attention. In *Behavioural models and the analysis of drug action* (ed. M.Y. Spiegelstein and A. Levy), pp. 89–107. Elsevier, Amsterdam.

Lyon, H.M., Kaney, S., and Bentall, R.P. The defensive function of persecutory delusions: evidence from attribution tasks. (In preparation.)

McCormick, D.J. and Broekema, V.J. (1978). Size estimation, perceptual recognition and cardiac rate response in acute paranoid and non-paranoid schizophrenics. *Journal of Abnormal Psychology*, **87**, 385–98.

McReynolds, P., Collins, B., and Acker, M. (1964). Delusional thinking and cognitive organisation in schizophrenia. *Journal of Abnormal and Social Psychology*, **69**, 210–12.

Magaro, P.A. (1984). Psychosis and schizophrenia. In *Theories of schizophrenia and psychosis. Nebraska symposium on motivation, 1983* (ed. W.D. Spaulding and J.K. Cole) pp. 157–230. University of Nebraska Press, Lincoln.

Magaro, P.A., Abrams, L., and Cantrell, P. (1981). The Maine scale of paranoid and non-paranoid schizophrenia: reliability and validity. *Journal of Consulting and Clinical Psychology*, **49**, 438–47.

Maher, B.A. (1974). Delusional thinking and perceptual disorder. *Journal of Individual Psychology*, **30**, 98–113.

Maher, B.A. (1988). Anomalous experience and delusional thinking: the logic of explanations. In *Delusional beliefs* (ed. T.F. Oltmanns and B.A. Maher) pp. 15–33. Wiley, New York.

Maher, B. and Ross, J.S. (1984). Delusions. In *Comprehensive handbook of psychopathology* (ed. H.E. Adams and P. Sutker) pp. 383–411. Plenum, New York.

Manschreck, T.C. (1979). The assessment of paranoid features. *Comprehensive Psychiatry*, **20**, 370–7.

Matussek, P. (1952). Studies in delusional perception. In *The clinical roots of the schizophrenia concept* (trans. J. Cutting and M. Shepherd (eds.) pp. 89–103, 1987). Cambridge University Press.

Maxwell, A.E. (1977). *Multivariate analysis in behavioural research.* Chapman and Hall, London.

Mayer-Gross, W., Slater, E., and Roth, M. (1969). *Clinical psychiatry.* Balliere, London.

Meehl, P.E. (1954). *Clinical versus statistical prediction: a theoretical analysis and a review of the evidence.* University of Minnesota Press, Minneapolis.

Meehl, P.E. (1964). A manual for use with a checklist of schizotypic signs. Unpublished manuscript. University of Minnesota.

Michotte, A. (1963). *The perception of causality.* Methuen, London.

Mill, J.S. (1872). *A system of logic ratiocinative and inductive* (8th edn). Longmans, Green, Reader & Dyer, London.

Milton, F., Patwa, V.K., and Hafner, R.J. (1978). Confrontation vs. belief modification in persistently deluded patients. *British Journal of Medical Psychology*, **51**, 127–30.

Mintz, S. and Alpert, M. (1972). Imagery vividness, reality testing and schizophrenic hallucinations. *Journal of Abnormal Psychology*, **79**, 310–16.

Moor, J.H. and Tucker, G.J. (1979). Delusions: analysis and criteria. *Comprehensive Psychiatry*, **20**, 388–93.

Mullen, P. (1979). Phenomenology of disordered mental function. In *Essentials of post-graduate psychiatry* (ed. P. Hill, R. Murray, and G. Thorley) pp. 25–54. Academic, London.

Murray, R.M., Lewis, S.W., Owen, M.J., and Foerster, A. (1988). Neurodevelopmental origins of dementia praecox. In *Schizophrenia: the major issues* (ed. P. McGuffin and P. Bebbington) pp. 73–90. Heinemann, London.

Mynatt, C.R., Doherty, M.E., and Tweney, R.D. (1977). Confirmation bias in a stimulated research environment: an experimental study of scientific inference. *Quarterly Journal of Experimental Psychology*, **30**, 395–406.

Neale, J.M. (1988). Defensive functions of manic episodes. In *Delusional beliefs* (ed. T.F. Oltmanns and B.A. Maher) pp.138–56. Wiley, New York.

Nelki, J. (1988). Making sense of a delusion of smell: a psychotherapeutic approach. *British Journal of Medical Psychology*, **61**, 267–75.

Nims, J.P. (1959). Logical reasoning in schizophrenia: the Von Domarus principle. Unpublished doctoral dissertation. University of Southern California.

Nisbett, R. and Ross, L. (1980). *Human inference: strategies and shortcomings of social judgement*. Prentice-Hall, Englewood Cliffs, NJ.

Nisbett, R.E. and Wilson, T.D. (1977). Telling more than we can know: verbal reports on mental processes. *Psychological Review*, **84**, 231–59.

O'Carroll, R. (1992). Neuropsychology of psychosis. *Current Opinion in Psychiatry*, **5**, 38–44.

Oltmanns, T.F. (1988). Approaches to the definition and study of delusions. In *Delusional beliefs* (ed. T.F. Oltmanns and B.A. Maher) pp. 3–12. Wiley, New York.

Oltmanns, T.F. and Maher, B.A. (ed.) (1988). *Delusional beliefs*. Wiley, New York.

Overall, J.E. and Gorham, D.R. (1962). The Brief Psychiatric Rating Scale. *Psychological Reports*, **10**, 799–812.

Paul, G.L. and Lentz, R.J. (1977). *Psychosocial treatment of chronic mental patients*. University Press, Cambridge, MA.

Payne, R.W. (1970). Disorders of thinking. In *Symptoms of psychopathology* (ed. C.G. Costello) pp. 49–94. Wiley, New York.

Pearce, J.M. and Hall, G. (1980). A model for Pavlovian learning: variations in the effectiveness of conditioned but not of unconditioned stimuli. *Psychological Review*, **87**, 532–52.

Persons, J.B. (1986). The advantages of studying psychological phenomena rather than psychiatric diagnosis. *American Psychologist*, **41**, 1252–60.

Phillips, J.P.N. (1970). A further type of Personal Questionnaire technique. *British Journal of Social and Clinical Psychology*, **9**, 338–46.

Phillips, J.P.N. (1977). Generalised Personal Questionnaire techniques. In *Dimensions of intrapersonal space*, Vol. 2 (ed. P. Slater). Wiley, Chichester.

Phillips, L.D. and Edwards, W. (1966). Conservatism in a simple probabilistic inference task. *Journal of Experimental Psychology*, **72**, 346–54.

Popper, K.R. (1959). *The logic of scientific discovery*. Hutchinson, London.

Price, H.H. (1934). Some considerations about belief. *Proceedings of the Aristotelian Society*, **35**, 229–52.

Quine, W.V.O. (1953). Two dogmas of empiricism. In *From a logical point of view*, pp. 20–46. Harvard University Press, Cambridge, MA.

Radley, A.R. (1974). Schizophrenic thought disorder and the nature of personal constructs. *British Journal of Social and Clinical Psychology*, **13**, 315–27.

Rattenbury, F.R., Harrow, M., Stoll, F.J., and Kettering, R.L. (1984). *The Personal Ideation Inventory: an interview for assessing major dimensions of delusional thinking*. Microfiche Publications, New York.

Raven, J.C. (1982). *The Mill Hill Vocabulary Scale: 1982 revision*. H.K. Lewis, London.

Reed, G. (1988). *The psychology of anomalous experience: a cognitive approach* (revised edn). Prometheus, Buffalo, NY.

Robertson, G. and Taylor, P.J. (1985). Some cognitive correlates of schizophrenic illnesses. *Psychological Medicine*, **15**, 81–98.

Ross, L. (1977). The intuitive psychologist and his shortcomings. In *Advances in experimental social psychology*, Vol. 10 (ed. L. Berkowitz) pp. 174–7. Academic, New York.

Ross, L. and Anderson, C.A. (1982). Shortcomings in the attribution process: on the origins and maintenance of erroneous social assessment. In *Judgement under uncertainty: heuristics and biases* (ed. K. Kahneman, P. Slovic, and A. Tversky) pp. 129–52. Cambridge University Press, New York.

Ross, L. and Lepper, M.R. (1980). The perseverance of beliefs: empirical and normative considerations. In *New directions for methodology of behavioral science: fallible judgement in behavioral research* (ed. R.A. Schweder and D. Fiske) pp. 129–52. Jossey-Bass, San Francisco.

Ross, M.B. and Magaro, P.A. (1976). Cognitive differentiation between paranoid and non-paranoid schizophrenics. *Psychological Reports*, **38**, 991–4.

Rudden, M., Gilmore, M., and Frances, A. (1982). Delusions: when to confront the facts of life. *American Journal of Psychiatry*, **139**, 929–32.

Russell, B. (1912). On induction. *The problems of philosophy*, ch. 6. George Allen & Unwin, London.

Russell, B. (1946). *A history of western philosophy*. George Allen & Unwin, London.

Sacks, M.H., Carpenter, W.T., and Strauss, J.S. (1974). Recovery from delusions. *Archives of General Psychiatry*, **30**, 117−20.

Salzinger, K. (1984). The immediacy hypothesis in a theory of schizophrenia. In *Theories of schizophrenia and psychosis. Nebraska symposium on motivation* (ed. W.D. Spaulding and J.K. Cole) pp. 231−82. University of Nebraska Press, Lincoln.

Scheibler, D. and Schneider, W. (1985). Monte Carlo tests of the accuracy of cluster analysis algorithms: a comparison of hierarchical and non-hierarchical methods. *Multivariate Behavioural Research*, **20**, 283−304.

Schlottman, A. and Shanks, D.R. (1992). Evidence for a distinction between judged and perceived causality. *Quarterly Journal of Experimental Psychology*, **44A**, 321−42.

Schmajuk, N.A. and Theime, A.E. (1992). Purposive behaviour and cognitive mapping: a neural network model. *Biological Cybernetics*, **67**, 1−10.

Schmajuk, N.A. and Tyberg, M. (1990). The hippocampal lesion model of schizophrenia. In *Neuromethods: animal models in psychiatry*, Vol. 19 (ed. A.A. Boulton, G.B. Baker, and M.T. Martin-Iverson). Heinemann, London.

Schmidt, G. (1940). A review of the German literature on delusion between 1914 and 1939. *Zentralblatt für die gesamte Neurologie und Psychiatrie*, **97**, 113−43. (In *The clinical roots of the schizophrenic concept* (trans. J. Cutting and M. Shepherd (ed.) pp. 104−34, 1987). Cambridge University Press.

Schneider, C. (1930). *Die Psychologie der Schizophrenen*. Thieme, Leipzig.

Schneider, K. (1959). *Clinical psychopathology* (trans. M.W. Hamilton). Grune & Stratton, New York.

Schwartz Place, E.J. and Gilmore, G.C. (1980). Perceptual organisation in schizophrenia. *Journal of Abnormal Psychology*, **89**, 409−18.

Sérieux, P. and Capgras, J. (1909). Misinterpretative delusional states. In *The clinical roots of the schizophrenia concept* (trans. J. Cutting and M. Shepherd (ed.) pp. 160−81, 1987). Cambridge University Press.

Shallice, T. (1988). *From neuropsychology to mental structure*. Cambridge University Press.

Shallice, T., Burgess, P.W., and Frith, C.D. (1991). Can the neuropsychological case study approach be applied to schizophrenia? *Psychological Medicine*, **21**, 661−73.

Shanks, D.R., Pearson, S.M., and Dickinson, A. (1989). Temporal contiguity and the judgement of causality by human subjects. *Quarterly Journal of Experimental Psychology*, **41B**, 139−59.

Shapiro, M.B. (1961). A method of measuring changes specific to the individual psychiatric patient. *British Journal of Medical Psychology*, **34**, 151−5.

Shapiro, M.B. and Ravenette, A.T. (1959). A preliminary experiment on paranoid delusions. *Journal of Mental Science*, **105**, 295−312.

Shepherd, G.W. (1984). Studies in the assessment and treatment of social difficulties in long-term psychiatric patients. Unpublished PhD thesis. Institute of Psychiatry, University of London.

Shiffrin, R.M. and Schneider, W. (1977). Controlled and automatic human information processing. II: Perceptual learning, automatic attending and a general theory. *Psychological Review*, **84**, 127–90.

Silverman, J. (1964). The problem of attention in research and theory of schizophrenia. *Psychological Review*, **71**, 352–79.

Slade, P.D. (1976). Towards a theory of auditory hallucinations: outline of a hypothetic four-factor model. *British Journal of Social and Clinical Psychology*, **15**, 415–23.

Slade, P.D. and Bentall, R.P. (1988). *Sensory deception: a scientific analysis of hallucination*. Croom Helm, London.

Slovic, P., Fischhoff, B., and Lichtenstein, S. (1977). Behavioural decision theory. *Annual Review of Psychology*, **28**, 1–39.

Snaith, R.P., Ahmed, S.N., Mehta, S., and Hamilton, M. (1971). Assessment of the severity of primary depressive illness. *Psychological Medicine*, **1**, 143–9.

Southard, E.E. (1916). On the application of grammatical categories to the analysis of delusions. *The Philosophical Review*, **25**, 424–55.

Spitzer, M. (1990). On defining delusions. *Comprehensive Psychiatry*, **31**, 377–97.

Spitzer, M. (1992). The phenomenology of delusions. *Psychiatric Annals*, **22**, 252–9.

Spitzer, R.L. and Endicott, J. (1977). *Schedule for affective disorders and schizophrenia — lifetime version (SADS-L)*. New York State Psychiatric Institute, New York.

Spitzer, R.L., Endicott, J., and Robins, E. (1975). Clinical criteria for psychiatric diagnosis and the DSM-III. *American Journal of Psychiatry*, **132**, 1187–92.

Spitzer, R.L., Endicott, J., and Robins, E. (1978). *Research diagnostic criteria for a selected group of functional disorders*. Biometrics Research, New York.

Squire, L. (1992). Memory and the hippocampus: a synthesis of findings with rats, monkeys and humans. *Psychiatric Review*, **99**, 195–231.

Stern, R.S. and Cobb, J.P. (1978). Phenomenology of obsessive–compulsive neurosis. *British Journal of Psychiatry*, **132**, 233–9.

Stocker, W. (1940). Quoted in Schmidt, G. *Zentralblatt for die Gesamte Neurologie und Psychiatrie*, **97**, 113–43.

Strauss, J.S. (1969). Hallucinations and delusions as points on continua function. *Archives of General Psychiatry*, **20**, 581–6.

Taylor, P.J., Garety, P.A., Buchanan, A., Reed, A., Wessely, S., Ray, K., Dunn, G., and Grubin, D. Delusions and violence. In *Violence and mental disorder: developments in risk assessment* (ed. J. Monahan and H.J. Steadman). Chicago University Press. (In press.)

Toone, B.K., Garralda, M.E., and Ron, M.A. (1982). The psychoses of epilepsy and the functional psychoses. *British Journal of Psychiatry*, **141**, 256–61.

Tversky, A. and Kahneman, D. (1982). Judgement under uncertainty: heuristics and biases. In *Judgement under uncertainty: heuristics and biases* (ed. D. Kahneman, P. Slovic, and A. Tversky) pp. 3–22. Cambridge University Press.

Volans, P.J. (1976). Styles of decision making and probability appraisal in selected obsessional and phobic patients. *British Journal of Social and Clinical Psychology*, **15**, 305–317.

Von Domarus, E. (1944). The specific laws of logic in schizophrenia. In *Language and thought in schizophrenia* (ed. J. Kasanin) pp. 104–13. University of California Press, Berkeley, CA.

Walkup, J. (1990). On the measurement of delusions. *British Journal of Medical Psychology*, **63**, 365–8.

Ward, J.H. (1963). Hierarchical grouping to optimise an objective function. *Journal of the American Statistical Association*, **58**, 236–44.

Wason, P.C. and Johnson-Laird, P.N. (1972). *Psychology of reasoning. Structure and content.* Batsford, London.

Watts, F.N., Powell, G.E., and Austin, S.V. (1973). The modification of abnormal beliefs. *British Journal of Medical Psychology*, **46**, 359–63.

Wessely, S., Buchanan, A., Reed, A., Everitt, B., Garety, P., Cutting, J., and Taylor, P. (1993). Acting on delusions (1): prevalence. *British Journal of Psychiatry*, **163**, 69–76.

Westermeyer, J. (1988). Some cross-cultural aspects of delusions In *Delusional beliefs* (ed. T.E. Oltmanns and B.A. Maher) pp. 212–29. Wiley, New York.

White, P.A. (1989). A theory of causal processing. *British Journal of Psychology*, **80**, 431–54.

White, P.A. (1990). Ideas about causation in philosophy and psychology. *Psychological Bulletin*, **108**, 3–18.

Williams, E.B. (1964). Deductive reasoning in schizophrenia. *Journal of Abnormal and Social Psychology*, **69**, 47–61.

Wing, J.K. (1988). Abandoning what? *British Journal of Clinical Psychology*, **27**, 235–8.

Wing, J.K., Cooper, J.E., and Sartorius, N. (1974). *The measurement and classification of psychiatric symptoms.* Cambridge University Press, Cambridge.

Winokur, G. (1978). Delusional disorder. In *Critical issues in psychiatric diagnosis* (ed. R.L. Spitzer and D.F. Klein) pp. 109–21. Raven, New York.

Winters, K.C. and Neale, J.M. (1983). Delusions and delusional thinking in psychotics: a review of the literature. *Clinical Psychology Review*, **3**, 227–53.

Winters, K.C. and Neale, J.M. (1985). Mania and low self-esteem. *Journal of Abnormal Psychology*, **94**, 252–90.

Wittgenstein, L. (1953). *Philosophical investigations* (trans. G.E.M. Anscombe, 1976). Blackwell, Oxford.

Wolfe, J.H., (1970). Pattern clustering by multivariate mixture analysis. *Multivariate Behavioural Research*, **5**, 329–50.

World Health Organization (1973). *The international pilot study of schizo-phrenia*. WHO, Geneva.

Zigler, E. and Glick, M. (1988). Is paranoid schizophrenia really camouflaged depression? *American Psychologist*, **43**, 284–90.

Zimbardo, P.G., Andersen, S.M., and Kabat, L.G. (1981). Induced hearing deficit generates experimental paranoia. *Science*, **212**, 1529–31.

Index